THE MENOPAUSE BOOK

THE MENOPAUSE BOOK

Barrie Anderson, M.D.
Elizabeth Connell, M.D.
Helen Singer Kaplan, M.D.
Nancy Kemeny, M.D.
Malkah Notman, M.D.
Johanna Perlmutter, M.D.
Natalie Shainess, M.D.
Mary Catherine Tyson, M.D.

edited by Louisa Rose

AN INFORMATION HOUSE BOOK

HAWTHORN BOOKS
A division of Elsevier-Dutton
New York

THE MENOPAUSE BOOK

Copyright © 1977 by Information House Books, Inc. Copyright under International and Pan-American Copyright Conventions. All rights reserved, including the right to reproduce this book or portions thereof in any form, except for the inclusion of brief quotations in a review. All inquiries should be addressed to Elsevier-Dutton, 2 Park Avenue, New York, New York 10016. This book was manufactured in the United States of America and published simultaneously in Canada by Clarke, Irwin & Company, Toronto and Vancouver.

Library of Congress Catalog Card Number: 79-9697

ISBN: 0-8015-4993-0 (cloth)
ISBN: 0-8015-4995-7 (paper)

1 2 3 4 5 6 7 8 9 10

CONTENTS

About the Authors — ix

Acknowledgments — xiii

Introduction — xv

1 WHAT IS MENOPAUSE? — 3

Stress • Menopause: An Emotional Problem • What Women Say about Menopause • The Physiology of Menopause • For Members of the Minority • Laying the Myths to Rest

2 TEMPORARY SYMPTOMS AND PERMANENT CHANGES — 18

Should You Ask Your Doctor? • Surgical Menopause • Vasomotor Instability • The Reason for Contraception • Abnormal Bleeding • Atrophic Changes • Osteoporosis • Depression • Changes In Physique • Other Changes • Regular Checkups

3 THE EMOTIONAL ELEMENT 35

The Stress Points • What We May Fear • How Society Takes Its Toll • When Problems Occur • Menopause for the Woman Alone • Where Are the Men of Yesteryear? • Living Well Alone, or Not So Alone • As the Twig Is Bent • Do You Need Psychotherapy? • What Kind of Therapy? • How to Find a Therapist • How to Know if You Have Chosen the "Right" Therapist • What to Do if You Are Troubled and Can't or Won't Seek Professional Help • Can You Talk to Your Children? • Reviving Friendships • The Virtues of Self-Indulgence • Intellectual Growth • Realistic Expectations • The Healthy Menopausal Woman

4 ESTROGEN: WHAT TO DO UNTIL THE RESULTS ARE IN 51

The Big Question • Discovery of the "Female Principle" • The Decisive Role of Estrogen • Estrogen and Puberty • The Other Sex Hormones • Measuring Estrogen Levels • Estrogen Production at Menopause and Even Beyond • How We Study the Side Effects of Drugs • Prospective Studies • Retrospective Studies • Evaluating the Risks • Risk Versus Benefit • The Studies Are Still Inconclusive • Many Factors • A Mutual Decision • Before You Take Estrogen • Who Should Take Estrogen • Who Should *Not* Take Estrogen • The Decision • How Much Estrogen? • What about Other Hormones? • What Kind of Estrogen? • How Do You Take It? • Follow-Up • The Responsible Physician

5 HYSTERECTOMY 72

Benign Conditions that *May* Require Hysterectomy • Cancerous and Precancerous Conditions of the Genital Tract • Preparation for Hysterectomy • Unnecessary Surgery

CONTENTS | vii

6 BREAST CANCER 99

Who Is at Risk • Estrogens and Breast Cancer Incidence • Detection • Self-Examination • Mammography • Other Types of Screening • Breast Biopsy • Staging • What Type of Surgery Is Best? • Lumpectomy • After Surgery • Prostheses • What Treatment Is Done after Surgery? • Endocrine Manipulation

7 SEX AT MENOPAUSE 112

Changes in Our Sexual Organs • Attractiveness • Making Sexual Choices • Choosing Celibacy • Choosing Marriage • Enriching Your Sex Life in Marriage • Choosing Alternatives to Marriage • The Basic Physiology of the Sex Act • Making Love to an Older Man • Stimulation Techniques • Impotence in Older Men • Sex and Fantasy • Touching • Masturbation • Sex Therapy • A Difficult Transition • Don't Fulfill a Negative Image

8 IS THERE A MALE MENOPAUSE? 130

Manifestations • Precipitants • Sexual Changes—Age of Onset • Family • Age • Men and Women • Sexual Therapy

9 HELPING NATURE: DIET, EXERCISE, AND COSMETIC SURGERY 144

Health Decisions at Menopause • Weight • Changes in Calorie Needs • Special Problems • Osteoporosis • Vitamin B Complex • How to Choose a Diet • Emotional Factors in Reducing • Finding the Right Diet • Why Exercise Now • Choosing Your Own Way to Exercise • Good Ways to Exercise in Company • Exercising on Your Own • Ten Aids for Successful Exercise • Hypertension • Relaxation • Cosmetic Surgery •

Your Body Image and Personality • Who Makes the Decision? • When Is It Beneficial? • What It Can and Cannot Do • Who Should Not Have Cosmetic Surgery • Improving Skin through Surgery • Hair • Skin Care • The Overall Goal

10 WOMEN TALK ABOUT MENOPAUSE — 172

Resource Directory — 201

Health Resources • Publications • Physical Well-Being • Beauty Care • Cancer and Surgery • Emotional Well-Being • Educational Resources • Employment Resources • Publications • General Resources • Reading List

Index — 247

ABOUT THE AUTHORS

"What Is Menopause"
    by LOUISA ROSE

Editor of *The Menopause Book*, Ms. Rose is a writer with an MFA from Sarah Lawrence. For two years she wrote the "Journal about Home" page for *The Ladies Home Journal* and for one year the "Health and Beauty" page. She has done medical writing for the Eli Lilly Company, and has had two plays produced in New York.

"Temporary Symptoms and Permanent Changes"
    by JOHANNA PERLMUTTER, M.D.

Dr. Perlmutter is a gynecologist who has worked as a gynecological consultant to the National Center for Family Planning in Washington, D.C. She is now Assistant Professor of Obstetrics and Gynecology at Harvard Medical School, and head of the section on human sexuality in the department of Obstetrics and Gynecology at Beth Israel Hospital. She has spoken on menopause and has written extensively on women's health problems.

"The Emotional Element"
    by NATALIE SHAINESS, M.D.

Dr. Shainess is a psychiatrist and psychoanalyst who practices in New York City. She was formerly Assistant Clinical Professor of Psychiatry at the New York School of Psychiatry and is now a member of the faculty of the William Alanson White Psychoanalytic Institute and Lecturer in Psychiatry at Columbia University College of Physicians and Surgeons. Her writing has appeared in various professional journals and in the anthology *Sisterhood Is Powerful*.

x | ABOUT THE AUTHORS

"Estrogen: What to Do until the Results Are In"
   by ELIZABETH CONNELL, M.D.

Dr. Connell is a gynecologist who also has received an American Cancer Fellowship. In 1972 and 1973 she was Associate Professor of Obstetrics and Gynecology at the College of Physicians and Surgeons and Director of Research and Development, Family Life Services, at the International Institute for the Study of Human Reproduction at Columbia University. In addition to writing numerous articles for the medical and lay press, she is now Associate Director for Health Sciences at the Rockefeller Foundation. She edited and coauthored *Hormones, Sex and Happiness* and has written a column for *Redbook* magazine.

"Hysterectomy"
   by BARRIE ANDERSON, M.D.

Dr. Anderson received her M.D. from the State University of New York at Syracuse in 1967 and then served an internship in surgery and a residency in obstetrics and gynecology. She was certified in obstetrics and gynecology in 1973 and then served two years as fellow in gynecologic oncology at the Tufts-New England Medical Center in Boston. Dr. Anderson is now assistant professor of obstetrics and gynecology at Tufts Medical School and is gynecologic oncologist at the New England Medical Center.

"Breast Cancer"
   by NANCY KEMENY, M.D.

Dr. Kemeny received her M.D. from the New Jersey College of Medicine and was trained at St. Luke's Hospital in New York City. She was certified in Internal Medicine in 1974. From 1974 to 1976 she held a fellowship in medical oncology at Memorial Hospital for Cancer and Allied Diseases in New York City and is now Assistant Attending in the Solid Tumor Service of the Department of Medicine there.

"Sex at Menopause"
   by HELEN SINGER KAPLAN, M.D.

Dr. Kaplan is Clinical Associate Professor of Psychiatry and in charge of student teaching of psychiatry at Cornell University College of Medicine, and head of the Human Sexuality Program at the New York Hospital-Cornell Medical Center, where she has developed and directs the clinic for brief treatment of sexual disorders. She also has a private practice in psychoanalysis and sex therapy. Dr. Kaplan has written for many professional journals and is the author of *The New Sex Therapy* and *The Illustrated Manual of Sexual Therapy*, and coeditor of *Progress in Group and Family Therapy*.

"Is There a Male Menopause?"
by MALKAH NOTMAN, M.D.

Dr. Notman is a psychiatrist who is now Associate Clinical Professor of Psychiatry at Harvard Medical School and has a practice in Brookline, Massachusetts. She is also a liaison-psychiatrist with obstetrics and gynecology at the Beth Israel Hospital in Boston. At the 1976 meeting of the American Psychiatric Association she led the panel, "A New Look at the Menopause and Mid-Life Years."

"Helping Nature: Diet, Exercise, and Cosmetic Surgery"
by MARY CATHERINE TYSON, M.D.

Dr. Tyson graduated from New York Medical College in 1937. She has been affiliated with Mt. Sinai Hospital since then. She was an intern and resident there, was chief of the Hematology Clinic, from 1950–1968, and taught medicine to nurses at the Mt. Sinai School of Nursing. In her private practice in New York City she specializes in internal medicine. Dr. Tyson is coauthor of two books: *The Psychology of Successful Weight Control* (with her husband, Dr. Robert Tyson) and *Good Food without Salt* (with Margaret Vaughn). She and her husband write a bimonthly medical-psychological column for *House and Garden* magazine.

ACKNOWLEDGMENTS

Many people worked to make this book as thorough and accurate as possible. Dian Smith, a tireless and dedicated coordinator, kept the information flowing and contributed valuable queries and comments. Beverly Savage worked hard to assemble the mass of practical information and recommended readings that make up our Resource Directory. Dana Kern Levenson, our Boston liaison, helped with research and interviews.

We are deeply grateful to those women who shared their experiences with us. It was difficult for some of them to talk about personal matters, but they felt it was important to let other women know that menopause can be a creative period in one's life.

Finally, special thanks are due to Dr. Henry Berman for his patient assistance in clarifying medical terminology and concepts.

LOUISA ROSE

INTRODUCTION

This is a book about menopause by a group of doctors and psychiatrists, all women, with special interest in and information about menopause.

As we write, there is no single handbook that is sufficiently comprehensive. We have tried to offer sound and thorough information on the subject, which is clear and factual without being either coy and oversimplified or ultratechnical. We've tried to answer for you all the questions we've been asked or that we would want to know ourselves: What symptoms can I expect and what do they mean? What can I do about them? What, if any, are the emotional problems I will face? What about my sexuality, my attractiveness, my vitality?

We have written this book for women who want intelligent and informed answers about menopause; for women who are no longer content to receive a pat on the head and a prescription for tranquilizers from their doctors when they complain of stress, anxiety, depression, or hot flashes. This is a book for women—and for the friends, children, husbands, and lovers of women—who face this potentially stressful period in their lives.

We have provided the most up-to-date information possible. Controversial subjects are presented here, especially in the chapters on hysterectomy, breast cancer, and estrogen replacement therapy, and we've tried as much to give help in sorting out the issues as to give our own advice and opinions. Each of these chapters will give you guidelines to use in making decisions based on your own personal needs and priorities. We have attempted to provide you with enough basic background information so that you may continue to ask intelligent questions of your own doctors.

We have tried to place menopause in context and show you that this is one more stage in the series of biological events that women experience.

In addition to specific material on medical problems, the book offers information on diet, exercise, and cosmetic surgery, as well as advice on sex for those who wish to revitalize this area of their lives. The resource directory is a specific guide to books, organizations, and services that can help you find a job, a doctor, or a sex counselor. We hope our book will enable you to head forth positively into the next years of your life, and that through reading the case histories and personal interviews with women who have already experienced menopause you will find that you share feelings and experiences with other women.

Finally, we trust that this book will help to put an end to myths and "old wives' tales," especially the notion that menopause is something to be dreaded or suffered. We also hope that it will help to change the outmoded child–parent relationship of patient to doctor. We would like to see the patient's role become a more active one, that of an informed and intelligent health services consumer.

Menopause is a normal change, not a tragedy, not an immense challenge, not a bad joke. Just a change. Some women welcome freedom from the menstrual cycle; some mourn the loss of their fertility. You'll discover through reading this book how complex and varied are women's responses. How will you handle menopause? If you are armed with the knowledge we give you, we think the choice is yours.

THE MENOPAUSE BOOK

1

WHAT IS MENOPAUSE?

What does menopause mean in our society? It is certainly not heralded with the "healthy" reaction we have recently learned is so important to demonstrate when a young girl gets her first period: "Now you are a woman." In fact, the opposite assumption is strongly at work. Now you are less than a woman—you won't be able to have babies. Your main task in life is over. Your sexuality is diminishing and your attractiveness is prey to each wrinkle, sag, and ounce of flab you accumulate. This process is accelerated in some women with the loss of estrogen; breasts tend to sag, the skin is drier, the vagina is less moist and elastic, hair thins. Lear proclaimed (admittedly in a different context) that "ripeness is all." But gone are the ample Venuses of Victorian or Rubenesque imaginings. Our present feminine ideal is reed-slim and smooth as an egg. Most women are too sensible to subscribe consciously to the trivialities of Miss America and the ad industry's feminine ideal. And yet so many women are on a perpetual diet, striving, not to create healthy bodies in keeping with their figure types but to conform to the present stereotype of beauty.

There is also a set of social prejudices about the menopausal woman, usually voiced behind the scenes—for example, in drug ads sent to doctors—but sometimes articulated publicly in high places. One of these was Washington, D.C., in 1970. Dr. Edgar Berman, who was Hubert Humphrey's personal physician and an appointee to the Democratic Party's Committee on National Priorities, raised a storm of protest when he attacked Congresswoman Patsy Mink's statement that she "wouldn't see anything wrong with a woman president." Dr. Berman raised the specter of women's alleged instability. "Suppose," he speculated, "that we had a menopausal woman president who had to make the decision on the Bay of Pigs. . . ." In fact, we had a president with Addison's disease (a deficiency disease of the adrenal glands), making what now may be regarded as a serious error in judgment. Betty Friedan, Shirley Chisholm, and even Dr. Berman's wife rose up in protest. Patsy Mink requested Dr. Berman's ouster from the committee. His response was to attack this as a "typical example of an ordinarily controlled woman under the raging hormonal imbalance of the periodical lunar cycle."

One might run through a list of ailments that have beset our male leaders but that never disqualified them from the burden of decision: Lincoln's melancholia, a symptom of a condition known as Marfan's syndrome; FDR's paralysis; LBJ's history of heart disease, and so on. Yet many employers combine with their general reluctance to hire older people a specific disinclination to hire women of menopausal age. They are considered too unstable to be competent, dependable workers. In discussing this, an employment counselor who specializes in placing older women noted that often when employers are persuaded to give such women a try, they are delighted with the result.

Many of our assumptions concerning women at menopause are based on the confused expectations that we have for women in general. These expectations are changing—slowly but truly. Yet, for those women who face menopause now, the changes offer only small comfort. Women who grew up in an era that approved of dependency, caring, homemaking, and child rearing as desirable feminine qualities, suddenly find themselves in a world proclaiming the virtues of assertiveness, self-expression, and self-sufficiency. Many women are unprepared to change and grow so drastically—or have been actively and systematically discouraged from doing so in the past.

"You can always go back to work when the children are grown up." In fact, many women have, and some have gained enormous satisfactions in finding new roles. But many other women have found themselves at age forty-five with enormous problems created by their earlier decision to stay home and mother: no marketable skills; no job history to adorn a resumé; no husband, through death or divorce;

and children with no place in their lives for mom. This is indeed a time of potential personal crisis, a crisis with no absolute relation to menopause except that *it's all happening at once.*

STRESS

Interestingly, there is no specific rating for menopause on the Holmes Stress Scale, a system of assigning levels of stress (from 1 to 100) to such events as divorce (73), change in recreation (19), and retirement (45). The inventors of this scale have attempted to quantify the amounts of stress produced by various life changes, both positive and negative. Those people with a rating of 300 points or more may experience actual physical symptoms as a result of too much change. For the woman experiencing menopause many of these changes tend to occur at the time that fluctuating hormone levels are already creating stress within her body. To get some idea of the amounts of stress experienced at this time of life, imagine a hypothetical woman. She is fifty years old—the average age at which menopause occurs. She is married and has two children. The younger has just left home for college; the older is married. She and her husband own their own home, with a mortgage of $8,000 yet to be paid. She has just resumed work as an executive secretary, work she had left to raise a family. Her boss is a finicky, demanding, and often irrational man. Because she works, she and her husband entertain at home less frequently and spend more time going out, either to the movies or for dinner. One of her closest friends has just died suddenly. She is trying to decide whether or not to take courses in business administration and go to her community college—a prospect that seems challenging and interesting to her. If we assign the stress "counts" to the various problems and changes in this woman's life we get the following:

Son or daughter leaving home	29
Gain of new family member	39
Mortgage under $10,000	17
Death of a close friend	37
Change in line of work[1]	35

[1]. This category of change must represent the woman's decision to return to work. Because of its innate sexism, this scale does not provide such a category.

Change in recreation	19
Change in financial state	38
Trouble with boss	23
Revision of personal habits	24

Without accounting for the stress of menopause, our hypothetical woman has a total of 261 stress points. For her, beginning course work might be just too much change for one year. How one reacts to stress is quite individual; some people are far more comfortable with change than others. But it is important to be aware that *you* might be under considerably more stress than you realize (positive changes can be as stressful as negative ones). This is typically a time of life filled with changes—children marry or go off to school, friends and family members die, marriages break up, women go back to work.

MENOPAUSE: AN EMOTIONAL PROBLEM

Much of the emotional instability of adolescence is attributed to changing hormone levels, yet the same reasoning is less often applied to explaining symptoms of menopause. Much more is made of the woman's emotional problems or the negative view society holds of her potential. Psychiatrists and psychologists have come up with explanations for the depression that accompanies menopause in a certain percentage of women. The authors of a recent book on menstruation, *The Curse*, trace the history of menopausal depression from the Victorian conviction that "during the menopause, a woman could expect to have mental problems." Among these problems are " 'morbid irrationality,' 'minor forms of hysteria,' melancholia and the impulses to drink spirits, to steal and perchance, to murder." The authors then go on to trace the unfortunate psychological stereotypes of the menopausal woman from Freud to the present. Freud characterized the menopausal woman as "quarrelsome and obstinate, petty and stingy . . . sadistic and anal-erotic." Helene Deutsch, psychoanalytic nemesis of the women's movement, viewed the menopause as the third edition of the infantile stage, the second being the menarche. In Deutsch's view the woman who becomes the servant of the species at the menarche emerges from menopause biologically useless. Erik Erikson perpetuates this image of a woman identified with her uterus in his analysis of menopause. To him, the menstrual period is an occasion for grief which becomes, at menopause, a "permanent scar." Morton Hunt, in *Her Infinite Variety*, characterized the menopausal woman as a silly, typically feminine creature who spent her days consulting astrologers and making "lemminglike migrations to see visiting movie stars." Women seeking therapy during their menopausal years might do well to find a therapist with a positive feminist orientation. Too many of those who are in the business of caring for our mental health hold outdated, extremely limited ideas of the possibilities that exist for women at this time in their lives. Yet there are therapists who recognize these possibilities. Analyst Clara Thompson sees menopause as a threat to women "who have postponed living until too late" and to women who only feel important "through the adulation of men." Here we have no deep-rooted psychological component of femininity, but a rather simple explanation in terms of life choices some women have made.

The authors of *The Curse* point to cultures where menopausal problems seem not to exist. "Most of the hazards of menopause are culturally induced. . . . The psychoanalyst George Devereaux has noted [among Mohave women]: In that society, the menopause is a sign of achievement; Mohave women are free to work, to flirt, and to be wise during their middle years."[2] Clara Thompson has concluded that "by far the greatest hazards of the menopause are psychogenical or culturally induced, and these are not so simply dispelled by a few pills. A psychiatrist working in China reported to me that she had never seen a menopausal psychosis in a Chinese woman. This she attributed to the fact that in China the older woman has a secure and coveted position."[3]

WHAT WOMEN SAY ABOUT MENOPAUSE

Very few studies have been made of how most of us think about, fear, hope for, or experience menopause. With all the speculation about the effects of the culture, the fears created by "old wives' tales," the intrinsic psychological problems, and the health problems that crop up, do we live in dread of the end of menstruation, do we feel

2. Janice Delaney, Mary Jane Lupton, and Emily Toth, *The Curse: A Cultural History of Menopause* (New York: E. P. Dutton, 1976), pp. 186–189.

3. Quoted in Paula Weideger, *Menstruation and Menopause: The Physiology and Psychology, the Myth and Reality* (New York: Knopf, 1976), p. 206.

that it will be an era of new freedom, or is it a matter of no importance? In one of the few studies made of women's opinions, Bernice Neugarten, a sociologist at the University of Chicago, questioned women of various ages, from twenty-one to sixty-five, to find out what they thought.[4] The results are illuminating. Women thirty and under held a far more negative view of menopause than those who were fifty-six and older, and who had presumably experienced it. For example, in the area of emotional problems, 48 percent of the young women agreed with the statement: "In truth, just about every woman is depressed about the change of life." Only 28 percent of the older group agreed. Twenty-eight percent of the young women agreed that "women lose their minds during the menopause," whereas 24 percent of the older group perceived this as a worry. The most startling differences are in the attitudes toward sexuality held by the various age groups. The older group seems to acknowledge more of an interest in sex than their younger sisters, daughters, and friends would grant them (there is a general tendency in our country to deny the sexuality of older people). A small group—8 percent—of the thirty and under age group agreed that "women would like to have themselves a fling at this time in their lives." Thirty-three percent of the thirty-one-to-forty-four-year-old women agreed; 32 percent of the forty-five-to-fifty-five-year-old women agreed; and 24 percent of those between fifty-six and sixty-five felt this to be true. Again, few (14 percent) of the younger women thought that women of menopausal age would be more interested in sex than before, while over a third (35 percent) of the women presumably experiencing menopause thought this was true. Another extremely interesting set of responses centers on the statement: "After the change of life a woman feels freer to do things for herself." Only 16 percent of the women under thirty agreed with this statement, as compared with a massive 74 percent of those women (forty-five to fifty-five) undergoing menopause. These women saw in menopause the chance to find greater personal freedom. Another statement in the area of self, "A woman gets more confidence in herself after the change of life," showed similar interesting discrepancies between younger and older groups. Twelve percent of those under thirty agreed, and 52 percent of those who were forty-five to fifty-five. Clearly, the older women who are

4. Bernice L. Neugarten and Ruth J. Kraines, "Menopausal 'Symptoms' in Women of Various Ages," *Psychosomatic Medicine*, March 27, 1965.

experiencing or have experienced menopause are far more positive about it than those who are younger—and remoter from this event. The younger women are afraid of the myths; the older women accept or welcome the reality.

In Europe, the International Health Foundation did a study of attitudes toward menopause of women aged forty-six to fifty-five. Over half the women questioned had completed menopause and another 23 percent were beginning to have signs of its approach. After personal interviews were conducted with 2,000 women—400 each from Belgium, France, Great Britain, Italy, and West Germany—the data for responses to each of thirteen statements about menopause were arranged and analyzed by country. The contrasts are fascinating.

Most of the statements were negative: for example, "Life becomes less interesting" or "The menopause brings physical upset." There were two negative statements with which a majority (over 50 percent) agreed: that menopause is psychologically upsetting and that it is physically upsetting. Other negative statements found the majority in disagreement. Of the five nationalities participating, the British women were the most positive; they disagreed in great numbers with negative ideas about menopause. For example, with the statement that "the menopause marks the beginning of old age," the British women were in active disagreement. Seventy-four percent disagreed as opposed to 37 percent of the Italians and 53 percent of the West Germans. When asked to take a position on whether "menopause means the end of attractiveness to men," the British disagreed even more strongly. Eighty-five percent did not think this to be true. The next largest group to take exception to this statement were the French women, 64 percent of whom disagreed. The differences in attitude from country to country suggest the powerful role culture plays in shaping our perceptions of our physiology. Are the British women responding with the traditional stiff upper lip? Or are they, as products of a culture that places more emphasis on individuality than on physical attractiveness, genuinely certain that they will continue to be interesting people, even when there's a drop in the estrogen supply?

THE PHYSIOLOGY OF MENOPAUSE

Everyone knows what menopause is. It is the cessation of menstrual periods, usually occurring in women forty-five to fifty-five, and it marks the end of reproduction. This is the usual definition and one that seems to wrap up the whole subject neatly. What more needs to be said? In fact, this description is inaccurate, for it makes menopause sound like an abrupt and sudden event, a dramatic "change of life." In fact, menopause is the final stage of a very gradual process.

Around the age of twenty-five, a woman's ovaries begin producing somewhat less estrogen. Estrogen is one of the two major female hormones (progesterone is the other) that have a number of important effects on a woman's body, including the establishment of the menstrual cycle; estrogen, in particular, has wide-ranging actions that affect many of her organ systems. Both hormones are produced by the ovaries in response to stimulation from other hormones sent from the pituitary, a gland situated just beneath the brain. A decrease in estrogen production can be detected as early as age twenty-five, but at first it is miniscule and for many years has no effect at all on a woman's menstrual periods. Somewhere between the ages of forty-five and fifty-five—although occasionally earlier or later—the estrogen produced by the ovaries is not sufficient to maintain normal monthly periods. Although some women stop menstruating quite suddenly, most experience a phase during which their periods are irregular and bleeding is either scantier or more copious than normal. This irregular phase may begin as long as five years before the actual menopause. At some point, the ovaries no longer respond to the hormones sent out by the pituitary, stop ripening eggs, and cease hormone production. There are no further periods—and menopause has occurred. (It is necessary, however, to continue to use birth control for a full year after the last period; not until then can you be sure that menstruation is really over.)

After menopause, small amounts of estrogen continue to be produced by a woman's adrenal glands—even though her ovaries are no longer functioning.

This seems simple, straightforward, and pretty unremarkable. But many important questions still to be answered lurk behind this factual explanation. Of all the mammals, why is the human female the only one that experiences a menopause? Other female animals continue to be fertile until death. Perhaps this is because animal young require a much shorter span of nurture before they achieve adulthood. Human babies with their protracted childhoods need prolonged mothering, and until recently women's average life-span has been considerably shorter than the present figure of seventy-eight for American women.

There are many other questions about menopause that have not been asked or examined until relatively recently, perhaps because most women just haven't been living that long. With the possibility of twenty-five to thirty years of adult life postmenopause, women are beginning to see that menopause and the years beyond present important problems. Greater amounts of time, energy, and money need to be spent on the study of women's physiology. Problems that have been assumed to be "neurotic" or socially induced may eventually turn out to have precise physical causes. At this point, researchers have not yet charted the exact chain of biochemical events that provoke menopause. What exactly causes the ovaries to shut down? What chemical message? Is there a more or less desirable hormonal balance in the female that allows for a smoother transition into menopause? Estrogen itself is not a simple substance but a group of several different estrogen compounds—estradiol, estriol, and estrone are the major ones—which may each have separate functions. One important task for research is to examine the role of estrogen stimulation in producing cancer of various types; eventually we may learn exactly which women ought to forego hormone replacement therapy after hysterectomy or menopause. For the moment, we do know sets of risk factors that identify those women who stand a greater than average chance of developing a cancerous growth. Another major area of investigation is the problem of osteoporosis, a thinning and weakening of the bones, which affects all women after menopause—some only mildly, some to a painful and debilitating degree. Estrogen is often used as therapy to slow down the loss of calcium and yet it will not remineralize bones. Can we look to a cure for this condition, or is it the inevitable progress of aging in a woman?

What any physiological definition of menopause fails to include is the cloud of myths, fears, and expectations that hovers over the term. We are women of a certain time and culture, heiresses to a set of images of ourselves that will determine our responses to what is an important stage of adult development. If the physiological definition of menopause seems simple, very little about the actual experience is, for menopause is a social, cultural, and personal emotional event in each woman's life. Every person can experience this natural event differently. Some researchers—sociologists, physicians, and psychologists—argue that the response to menopause is largely a question of individual *psychological* makeup. If you are physically healthy, stable, and productive, and have a positive self-image, your menopause will be relatively easy. If you are neurotic, dependent, undergoing some personal or marital crisis, or chronically depressed, and do not accept your own womanhood—then you are in for a rough time. Until fairly recently, this view was widely accepted; but women have begun to question it, and some of their doctors now have strong doubts. Each woman has an individual hormone balance that plays a prominent part in her response. Women whose endocrine glands gradually stop producing estrogen will experience fewer and milder symptoms than women with abrupt variations in hormone levels. It is interesting that women who have undergone "surgical menopause" (removal of the ovaries) and consequently have an abrupt cessation of estrogen production consistently report some severe menopausal symptoms. Yet these are often women in their thirties, women with full nests, with youthful bodies and faces, and quite a few years to go before they must confront "the crisis of middle age."

What we all need to fight against is the tendency bred in ourselves, fostered by the society we live in and reinforced by the physicians who are in the business of caring for our bodies, that women's complaints are just that—complaints, the products of childlike, trivial, neurotic minds, to be dismissed with a pat on the back, a prescription for a potentially addictive drug such as Valium, or an ill-considered course of estrogen replacement therapy prescribed without a thorough physical evaluation and a full discussion with the patient of the risks and benefits of the potent drug she is about to take.

Doctors' estimates vary, but somewhere between 10 and 30 percent of menopausal women have symptoms serious enough to cause them to seek medical advice. Some of them may have only mild symptoms, of course, but those women who experience severe symptoms deserve careful and thorough attention. They are feeling real discomfort; they are not merely "neurotic" or "hysterical."

The International Health Foundation study cited earlier undertook an examination of the range of symptoms experienced by menopausal women. At first, the respondents were asked to name any complaints they had experienced which they believed to be connected with menopause. Hot flushes were mentioned by 37 percent, headaches by 19 percent, excessive sweating by 18 percent, and nervousness by 17 percent. When the women were shown a list of symptoms, many more answered that they had indeed experienced them. Possibly they had never thought of connecting the symptoms on the list with menopause.

The symptoms most commonly reported by women in this age group were hot flushes, tiredness, nervousness, and excessive sweating. Tiredness and nervousness may be allied—the result not of menopause but of being awakened by night sweats. The table below, reprinted from the International Health Foundation Study, shows the extent to which these women experienced menopausal symptoms—and during which phase of menopause they were most likely to occur.

	Respondents still experiencing regular menstrual cycles	Respondents experiencing irregular cycles	Respondents in the post-menopause
	%	%	%
Hot flushes	20	35	35
Tiredness	30	50	45
Nervousness	29	48	44
Excessive sweating	15	42	48
Headaches	26	44	40
Sleeplessness	20	35	35
Depression	17	36	34
Irritability	20	38	29
Joint pains	17	25	29
Dizziness	10	29	27
Palpitations	15	27	27
Lassitude	15	28	22
Pins and needles	13	27	23
Muscle pains	12	25	24
Breathlessness	11	19	20
Impatience	10	20	16
Other complaints	6	16	11
No complaints	37	6	9

From: International Health Foundation, *The Menopause: A Study of the Attitudes of Women in Belgium, France, Great Britain, Italy and West Germany*, p. 31.

The most recent survey of women's attitudes toward menopause was undertaken by The Boston Women's Health Book Collective to gather information for a revision of the now famous *Our Bodies, Ourselves.*[5] Two thousand questionnaires were sent out; 484 were completed and returned. Fifty-two percent of the answers came from women between the ages of forty-one and sixty. About two-thirds of this group worked outside the home, and the authors speculate that many of the positive responses from these menopausal and postmenopausal women are the result of their active role in the world.

About two-thirds of menopausal and postmenopausal women reported hot flashes. Here, as in Europe, this is a reliably common symptom. About two-thirds of this group who had either experienced or were now experiencing menopause "felt neutral or positive about the changes they experienced." The remaining third were "clearly negative." Interestingly, loss of child-bearing ability was not a reported concern. (Much of the psychoanalytical theorizing about menopause is based on the supposed blow this represents to a woman's identity.) Instead, the survey showed that 90 percent felt either positive or neutral. The authors feel that this apparent discrepancy between psychological theory and reported fact may be due to the nature of the group that responded, and if they are right, it is a lesson to women of all ages. "Although our culture has attached great importance to a woman's ability to reproduce, most women in our sample were not upset by the end of menstruation. Possibly this reflects the fact that for these women childbearing ability was only part of their self-image. After menopause they were able to value (and had the opportunity to develop) their talents and capacities beyond childbearing. Perhaps for most of these women it was a simple matter to accept this biological change as an inevitable and natural part of aging."[6]

In preparing this book, we have talked to many women about their experiences with menopause. Some declined to be interviewed; others were glad to share their experiences with other women. All expressed a desire to be anonymous and this has been respected. The essentials of their life experiences and feelings about menopause are all true but their identities have been fictionalized.

5. The Boston Women's Health Book Collective, *Our Bodies, Ourselves* (New York: Simon and Schuster, 1976).
6. Ibid., p. 335.

Later, in chapter 9, you may read extended verbatim accounts of the experiences of eight women. They speak in their own words. Here, I would like to share my impressions of what they were saying and the importance it has for women who are beginning or about to begin this period of their lives. The most profound impression I had was that menopause is an entirely individual experience. Even though quite a large number of women will experience one or more hot flashes—perhaps hundreds—each person has a distinct style of dealing with them. Some women find them annoying, some find them embarrassing. Others only recall their occurrence after careful questioning.

One woman claimed to have never experienced any symptoms at all. (It had to be pointed out that the palpitations she occasionally had might be connected with menopause.) This woman doesn't understand what all the fuss is about—menopause is a trivial event. "There's no point in interviewing me," she said. "I couldn't be of any use to you because I never experienced anything at all." Other women had difficult and painful problems. Often, they were told by their doctors, "You're just going through menopause." Very few of the women interviewed for this book were given the kind of medical information and support that might have helped them. Either they were given estrogen without any discussion of side effects or risks or they were told that the doctor did not believe in giving "a lot of medication."

Many of these women, though, did not want to be responsible health consumers. They viewed the doctor as a paternal figure who would tell them what was good for them to know. This is an attitude that is beginning to change—and the sooner the better. There are areas of health care where it is vitally important for women to seek full knowledge of alternatives, to know what is normal and what is a danger sign, and to know when it is important to ask for a second opinion. For example, certain kinds of vaginal bleeding, including any bleeding that occurs after menopause, should be reported immediately to a gynecologist. Although usually resulting from benign problems, abnormal bleeding may occasionally be a sign of cancer—and here early detection is vital. Cancer is not always hopeless; it is often curable. Women who are experiencing symptoms of menopause—flushes and sweats—which make them totally miserable do have the option of taking estrogen. They need to discuss with their doctors whether the risks involved outweigh the benefits. Short-term, low-dosage estrogen therapy is still considered acceptable and may make the lives of many women more bearable during a trying time. Those women who have a relatively easy menopause are fortunate. They are also in the majority.

FOR MEMBERS OF THE MINORITY

While it is comforting to know before menopause that you stand a good chance of experiencing few difficulties, it is small comfort if you are one of the minority who has a difficult time. One woman had a hysterectomy at about the time she was beginning to experience menopausal symptoms. "I had headaches and I was really upset because I wanted to feel good. But what I noticed I had was really a cranky kind of thing. Strange funny feelings." She was a woman who had sailed through five pregnancies, and described herself as happily married with a supportive family.

Another woman, mother of three grown children and busily engaged in a demanding and exciting new job, found that she was experiencing hot flashes on an hourly basis. "Oh, they were nothing. I just got through them," was her response. Still, they were troublesome enough for her to try estrogen therapy. It is important to acknowledge that those women who have difficulty with menopause have real complaints, for which they deserve the same help and sympathy anyone with a physical complaint is entitled. They are not malingerers or neurotics.

LAYING THE MYTHS TO REST

A great deal that is damaging to our self-esteem as women is passed off as expert knowledge by misinformed and dangerously biased men. An example of this is the discussion of menopause in *Everything You Always Wanted To Know About Sex* (but Were Afraid to Ask)* by David Reuben, M.D. After ascribing menopause to a "defect in evolution" he goes on to characterize estrogen as "the entire basis of femininity" and as "responsible for that strange mystical phenomenon, the feminine state of mind." Contrary to much current research on female sexuality, he has ascribed sexual desire to "the ebb and flow of estrogenic hormone during the menstrual cycle. . . . Once the ovaries stop, the very essence of being a woman stops." Here, woman is reduced to ovary. The fact that large numbers of women report an *increase* in sexual drive near or during menstruation at a time when estrogen levels are at their lowest, and that many women report an increase in sexual drive *after* menopause, seems to have escaped Dr. Reuben.

The Menopause Book is an attempt to lay the myths and fears and prejudices to rest, to deal with the facts of menopause, to attend to the problems, and to encourage the woman who is arriving at this "change of life" to assert her need for good medical advice, and for support from family, husband, lover, or friends. More and more women are beginning to perceive this as a time of great growth and as an opportunity to explore their own individuality.

2
TEMPORARY SYMPTOMS AND PERMANENT CHANGES

How does a woman know that she is about to begin the series of changes that lead to menopause? What physical symptoms will she feel and what signs will her body give that indicate this phase of life is under way? These are the questions that we will try to answer as fully as possible in this chapter. Menopause is for all of us a highly variable and individual experience. What is a sign and what is a symptom?

The word *menopause* refers to a very specific period of time: the end of menstruation. Although we tend to associate menstruation with the workings of the uterus, what really happens is that the ovaries gradually stop functioning. Menopause is the outcome when they no longer produce hormones that will trigger ovulation. Doctors can only make a definite diagnosis of "menopause" after an entire year has elapsed during which there is no vaginal bleeding. At this point, menopause is considered to have occurred, and women can stop using birth control methods.

The years leading up to the actual menopause are called the *premenopausal* years. Although there is no way to define the onset of this era precisely, women gradually become aware that changes are occurring in their bodies. After menopause has been reached, women are considered to be *postmenopausal*. The years encompassed by premenopause, menopause, and postmenopause are referred to by various terms: the perimenopausal years, the *climacteric*, and the *change of life*.

SHOULD YOU ASK YOUR DOCTOR?

Doctors estimate that about 80 percent of women will experience some symptoms and therefore will be aware that they are going through menopause. Most complaints, however, are minor ones and only an estimated 25 to 30 percent of women are made sufficiently uncomfortable by their symptoms to seek medical attention. Since each woman's response is individual, it is difficult to predict whether or not someone will develop problems. Unfortunately, many physicians are uncomfortable when patients ask questions, because they simply don't know the answers. Those who are persistent enough to continue asking questions about their health, may find their queries falling on deaf ears.

> L. J. is a forty-eight-year-old woman who has specifically made an appointment to see the doctor because of her irregular light menses and the sudden awareness of intense perspiration at odd times of the day. At the physician's office, she starts to tell the doctor about her concerns, and he promptly tells her not to worry and starts questioning her about her heart and lungs. At the completion of her physical examination, she is told that all is well and she is in perfect health. She is dismissed from the office before she can reiterate her questions and concerns.

If you are in L. J.'s situation—unable to broach the subject of menopause—then you may never seek or get the professional help you deserve. You have the right to expect your doctor to spend time answering your questions in an honest, direct way. During your annual examination, ideally your physician will ask a number of questions about your general health and take the initiative in asking specifically about menopause.

Information about the severity of complaints or symptoms is limited and doctors need to know much more about this area. What we do know is that the spectrum of symptoms women experience ranges from no problems at all through minimal problems to an array of very severe, discomforting symptoms that interfere with day-to-day functioning.

Following is an example of a woman with very minor symptoms:

P.T. is a fifty-one-year-old woman who stopped having periods a year ago. Prior to that time, she noted that her menstrual flow had been getting scantier and that her periods occurred less frequently, until they finally ceased. Her only other symptom of menopause (of which she was aware) was that every once in a while she would notice being fairly warm. She went about her daily activities with no interruptions. Finally, she asked her doctor when she was going to develop menopausal symptoms and was pleasantly surprised to learn that she had already passed through what would have been the most difficult period of time and probably would have no further problems.

In contrast to this very easy menopause is the case of a woman who has experienced great difficulty.

H. J. is a forty-five-year-old woman who is still menstruating regularly but has been having hot flashes for the past two years. Her complaints are extreme tiredness and fatigue so severe that she has difficulty getting up in the morning and going to work. She is somewhat depressed and concerned about how she can continue her normal daily schedule. She has developed severe headaches that are unrelieved by her usual medications. The hot flashes cause her clothing to become so drenched that she has to change her outfits at least two or three times a day. She is so disturbed by this symptom that she no longer leaves the house for any reason.

What kind of menopause will *you* have?

Doctors do not yet have accurate enough diagnostic tools to predict how any individual woman will react to menopause, what her symptoms will be, or how severe. Neither body size nor contour, physical characteristics, age at onset of menstruation, length of periods, nor degree of menstrual discomfort gives any reliable indication. Until fairly recently, all of the symptoms that menopausal women complained about were labeled "emotional disturbance." We now have sufficient knowledge of the physical origins of symptoms so that those who experience symptoms are no longer sent first to a psychiatrist and only subsequently to a gynecologist.

SURGICAL MENOPAUSE

For some women, premenopausal changes may be rather abrupt. If a woman's ovaries are removed (ovariectomy or oophorectomy), her periods will cease at once and the onset of menopause will occur with little or no opportunity for the gradual premenopausal adjustment to hormonal changes. This sudden rapid change in hormonal balance sometimes makes women quite uncomfortable until their bodies can reacclimate to the new state. The degree of discomfort is a great variable and cannot be predicted ahead of time. (Radiation treatment for malignancies may also cause the ovaries to stop functioning and thus create an abrupt menopause.) On the other hand, surgical loss of the uterus, while it also results in the sudden cessation of menstruation, does not nececcarily reul in menopause. The word *hysterectomy* is sometimes used with great lack of precision. Total hysterectomy refers only to the removal of the uterus and cervix and does not stipulate whether or not the ovaries have been left in place. The uterus is an end organ, which means that it responds to hormonal stimulation but it does not produce or affect hormonal balance in any way. Even though there is no uterus and therefore no further vaginal bleeding, menopause, which is a *hormonal* change, does not occur unless the ovaries, too, have been removed. In fact, women who have equated "hysterectomy" with menopause have been quite surprised many years later when they have begun to experience menopausal symptoms; their ovarian function beginning to diminish in the normal course of events.

> B. D. is a forty-eight-year-old woman who had a hysterectomy at age thirty for fibroids. She was told at the time of her procedure that she had had a total hysterectomy and everything had been removed. She had not been given any hormonal therapy and had assumed that she had gone through her change of life, although she never had any symptoms. She no longer had the cyclic mood changes she had experienced before the hysterectomy and was no longer bleeding vaginally. At forty-seven, she began to have hot flashes and night sweats. Thinking she had already had a surgical menopause, she was totally perplexed as to what these were but never thought to ask her gynecologist. She was convinced that

there was something radically wrong but did not seek medical attention for over a year, fearing that the doctors really might find something wrong with her. When she finally went to a doctor because the hot flashes had become unbearable, she felt very foolish when she learned that her symptoms were menopausal.

If all of the ovarian tissue is removed at the time of surgery, then women begin to have menopausal symptoms. If however, even a small amount of ovarian tissue remains, it will continue to produce estrogen until such time as a woman would naturally go through her menopause. There is, at present, no evidence that equates the amount of ovarian tissue with the onset of menopause. Small pieces of ovarian tissue seem to work as effectively as an entire ovary.

As each of the difficulties that have been associated with the menopause are described in the following pages, you will realize how much remains to be learned about how and why the body functions as it does. We are now beginning to understand some of the hormonal changes that occur during the climacteric, but what exactly triggers this sequence of hormonal changes is as yet unknown. Although we discuss waning estrogen levels and loss of progesterone due to lack of ovulation, these are not the only factors causing menopausal symptoms.

VASOMOTOR INSTABILITY

One of the most common symptoms and one of the earliest signs of approaching menopause is a vasomotor symptom, commonly called a hot flush or hot flash. A vasomotor symptom occurs as a result of the dilation or contraction of tiny blood vessels in response to messages from the nerves. Women have described a hot flash as the sudden onset of a feeling of warmth that pervades the upper part of the body. In association with this, you may develop a flushed face and find patchy red areas on your chest, back, shoulders, and upper arms. The flushes may then be followed by profuse perspiration, which will leave you with a cold, clammy sensation as your body temperature readjusts to its surroundings. Hot flushes occur very sporadically and may originate several years before there is any objective evidence that you are nearing menopause. Hot flushes are thought to be a sign of waning estrogen levels. As the actual time of menopause approaches, they may become more frequent and more noticeable.

The sensations vary from woman to woman and also from one episode to another. They may seem very mild or very uncomfortable and may last from a few seconds to as long as half an hour, perhaps longer.

If you are a woman who works outside the home, it may be embarrassing in the middle of a meeting or during an important decision or discussion suddenly to turn red in the face, have the need to start fanning yourself, and have difficulty breathing because of the intense warmth that you feel. Your anxiety may increase and prolong your discomfort. Although these attacks are probably caused by normal hormonal imbalances, they can be precipitated by stress and excitement.

One way of minimizing the problem is to learn to dress differently so that you can acclimate yourself to sudden changes in body temperature. For example, a sleeveless dress with a jacket that may be shed at a moment's notice allows you to strip and redress unobtrusively, maintain your decorum, and periodically adapt yourself to your body changes and to your surroundings.

When these flashes, flushes, episodes of perspiration, or attacks—whichever you wish to call them—occur at night, they can disturb your sleep. In extreme cases, the perspiration may be so profuse that clothes and bed linens need to be changed. This may be unsettling to you and may affect the entire household.

The hot flash is a consequence of the ovary's failing production of estrogens. But there must be other factors. Curiously, estrogen levels are very low in patients with stress amenorrhea (no menses under tension) or anorexia nervosa (a psychiatric condition associated with loss of weight and loss of menses), but hot flashes do not occur. FSH (follicle stimulating hormone), certain chemicals called releasing factors, and other hormones that are produced by the hypothalamus or pituitary glands may play a role in producing hot flashes.

Flashes, if they appear, will reach a maximum when estrogen dips to its minimum level, just about the time of actual cessation of menses. As your body readjusts itself to the lowered hormonal level, hot flashes will diminish in number and intensity and will eventually disappear completely. It is impossible to predict the length of time over which hot flashes will occur, but on the average, you can expect to experience them for about five years.

Since the hot flash results from a specific hormonal change, it is one of the few manifestations of menopause that is completely amenable to treatment. Usually, an estrogen preparation is given in a dose sufficient to relieve symptoms. Because of the serious questions recently raised about the safety of estrogen, you should discuss the pros and cons of the use of this medication with your physician. Estrogen therapy should continue only so long as you really need it. It should then gradually be tapered off. Abrupt cessation of treatment will generally intensify your symptoms, which is why gradual withdrawal of medication is necessary. If you are taking estrogen and want to stop using it, you need to discuss your plan for doing so with your doctor.

THE REASON FOR CONTRACEPTION

The term *menstruation*—strictly speaking—refers to the cyclical vaginal bleeding associated with the ovulatory cycle. But women do not necessarily ovulate every month. Ovulatory cycles (in which an egg is released) are few in number just after puberty, rise to a maximum in the twenties, and gradually diminish again until the menopause is reached. Usually you are unaware that ovulation is no longer occurring since you still experience monthly vaginal bleeding at more or less regular intervals. Some women claim that it is easy to tell the difference between ovulatory and *an*ovulatory (no egg released) bleeding. The latter, they say, is usually painless and the former is associated with some discomfort and varying premenstrual symptoms, such as bloatedness and irritability. In reality, it is frequently very difficult to distinguish between the two types of cycles and most women are unaware of whether or not ovulation has taken place.

As estrogen levels wane, the most typical bleeding pattern is a shortening of the duration of your period and a lengthening of the interval between periods. Eventually, there is no further bleeding; menopause, the complete cessation of menses, has occurred. This natural progression of delayed and missed menses coupled with light bleeding can be very anxiety-provoking if pregnancy is a possibility for you. Although ovulation during this period of time is very sporadic and infrequent, it can and does occur. Pregnancies have been re-

TEMPORARY SYMPTOMS AND PERMANENT CHANGES | 25

ported in women in their fifties. It is therefore imperative that you continue to use contraception until you have spent an entire year without a period. For women approaching menopause, the safest methods of birth control are the diaphragm and the condom. Another safe choice, of course, is sterilization. The IUD is not recommended because it can cause irregular bleeding and necessitate investigation into the cause of the abnormal bleeding. The latest studies on oral contraceptives show a definite increase in heart disease and heart attacks in women over forty who take the pill. The rhythm method of birth control is even less effective during the menopausal era than at other times because of the irregularity of menstrual periods.

ABNORMAL BLEEDING

This time of life can be trying because it is difficult for you to know exactly what "normal" bleeding is. Instead of scant, infrequent bleeding, you may note that your periods are heavier. At times, small clots may be passed. Once in a while, the bleeding may be prolonged and even profuse. In addition, some bleeding or spotting may occur midcycle or after intercourse. It is imperative that you consult your gynecologist. Even though most often a specific cause for the bleeding cannot be found, you must not assume it is merely a menopausal symptom that can be discounted. Occasionally, a serious problem may be the cause.

If no specific cause for the abnormal bleeding is found, it is usually called "dysfunctional" and thought to be the result of a hormonal imbalance caused by lack of ovulation. Progesterone produced as a result of ovulation, matures the lining of the uterus, the endometrium, so that it is shed at the time of menstruation. In the absence of adequate progesterone, an irregular shedding of the endometrium may occur and may result in an irregular bleeding pattern. Several benign conditions also cause abnormal bleeding: cervical polyps, endometrial polyps, cervicitis (inflammation of the cervix), and vaginal infections. These benign conditions usually respond to appropriate therapy. Doctors are concerned about the small number of women who may have either a cervical or a uterine malignancy for which early detection may mean a successful cure. Often, the only early symptom of such a malignancy is abnormal bleeding.

In order to diagnose the cause of abnormal bleeding, your doctor will take a thorough history and do a physical examination which includes a Papanicolaou (Pap) smear. A Pap smear, properly performed, is a valuable diagnostic tool. This test may show the presence of infections such as monilia, of infections such as trichomonas, of inflammation of the cervix—and more importantly, is an indicator of premalignant or malignant cell changes in the cervix. If these measures do not pinpoint the cause of the bleeding (and they often do not), an operative procedure may be necessary. Usually a D & C (dilatation and curettage is required. This procedure involves dilating the cervix and doing a curettage (or scraping of the endometrium). Sometimes, the D & C will correct the bleeding pattern even when a specific cause for the problem is not found.

It is really very difficult to define what is an absolutely normal bleeding pattern during the menopausal years. In general, if your vaginal bleeding is the same as it has been in the past or somewhat scantier than usual, this is a normal and reassuring pattern. Bleeding which occurs at regular intervals or becomes less frequent is also normal. In rare cases, your bleeding pattern will appear to be perfectly normal and then suddenly cease. Under these circumstances you may fear pregnancy, but it is usually the normal onset of menopause. Having a routine urinary pregnancy test may increase your anxiety, as false positive results can occur. The newer blood tests for pregnancy are helpful in distinguishing between the hormonal changes of menopause and pregnancy, and this is an area in which your physician should be able to help you.

After you have stopped having periods for at least one year, any form of bleeding is abnormal. Malignancy is the gravest concern, but it is not the only cause of bleeding. Vaginitis (inflammation) and atrophy (thinning) of the vaginal lining may cause this bleeding. Also, inappropriate and prolonged use of hormones without proper physician supervision may be responsible. Any bleeding, spotting, or staining that occurs after your menopause needs to be promptly investigated by a doctor.

ATROPHIC CHANGES

Nearly all of the tissues including the skin undergo atrophic (shrinking or thinning) changes with advancing years. This process is part of aging. Some of these changes are directly related to loss of hormones while others are independent of the endocrine system. It is sometimes difficult to separate the two causes. Loss of elasticity and sagging are probably not hormonally dependent. Dryness, loss of lubrication, and thinning of the tissues, on the other hand, are probably secondary to the loss of hormones.

After menopause, the cervix (mouth of the womb) no longer produces mucus and the uterus itself gradually shrinks in size. This process does not usually cause any difficulty, and you will probably be unaware of these changes. Aside from the fact that you will no longer be able to bear a child, these particular alterations need not affect your femininity and your sense of yourself as a sexual human being.

The mucosa (lining) of the vagina gradually becomes thinner, dryer, and less elastic. Your vagina may not stretch to accommodate your partner's penis as readily as when you were younger. If you have been enjoying an active sex life while going through your menopause, you may not even be aware of these changes. Occasionally, you may notice that you do not lubricate as well or as rapidly as you used to and that intercourse may become somewhat painful. This is a problem you should definitely discuss with your doctor. If this should occur, local estrogen cream or simply K-Y jelly may be helpful. If you are also having other symptoms of menopause that are due to lack of hormones, oral medication may be your doctor's recommendation. If you did not have intercourse while you went through your menopause and for several years thereafter, you may experience discomfort if you resume your sex life. The vagina tends to shrink if it is not kept dilated by intercourse during this critical period of time. Estrogens, applied locally or taken systemically, will aid in the restoration of the vaginal mucosa. Needless to say, the best stimulus for good lubrication and dilatation of the vagina is to make sure you are "turned on." You may need a long period of sexual foreplay to allow adequate lubrication to occur, and this added time will enhance your own and your partner's pleasure. In the absence of adequate lubrication, penile entry into the vagina may cause pain, burning sensations, and tearing or bleeding of the vaginal tissues.

> L. J. is a fifty-five-year-old woman who has been a widow for ten years. She went through menopause at the age of forty-eight with minimal discomfort and remained free of any symptoms for four

years. But when she recently met a man and began a love affair, her first attempt at intercourse created so much pain and discomfort that she immediately sought medical attention. Use of local estrogen cream and some counseling on sex techniques allowed her to resume sexual activity, and both partners now enjoy satisfying and pleasurable sex.

Before we leave the vagina, there is one other problem that can develop postmenopausally, namely vaginal discharge. The medical term for this condition is senile vaginitis. Loss of hormones, changes in the vaginal tissues, and dryness of the area may lead to inflammation and infection. Sometimes vaginal creams and preparations alleviate the problem temporarily. But for a woman who is plagued by repeated infections, topical estrogen cream is usually beneficial. Again, consultation with your physician is necessary to determine what is the appropriate therapy for you.

After menopause, along with the atrophy of the other genital tissues, the labia majora (the larger skin folds) will also gradually shrink in size. Thus the urethra and vagina are more exposed to abrasions and irritations from panties, panty hose, and girdles, because this sensitive area no longer has the natural covering of the labia to protect it.

In addition, minor anatomical changes may occur as the vagina shortens and shrinks. In some cases, the urethral meatus (opening of the urethra) may be pulled into and become part of the outer portion of the vagina causing urethral inflammations and urinary tract infections. This situation may be aggravated by intercourse causing a mechanical irritation which can give you urinary symptoms even when no infection is evident. Women with urinary symptoms should seek medical attention for this problem.

The thinning of the tissues around the vagina, urethra, bladder, and rectum sometimes leads to marked relaxation and prolapse (falling) of these structures into the vagina. The technical terms for these problems are *urethrocele* (descent of the urethra into the vagina), *cystocele* (bladder descent), and *rectocele* (rectal descent). A sensation of heaviness in the vaginal area or the feeling that tissue is protruding from the vagina may indicate what is happening. In extreme cases and with marked relaxation, even the cervix and uterus may prolapse into the vagina and may in fact descend out beyond the vaginal opening. Some sort of correction is necessary. A pessary (a rubber doughnut-shaped object) may be inserted into the vagina in an attempt to restore the organs to their original position. The tissues may be so relaxed that it may be impossible to get a good fit with a pessary. Moreover, pessaries are only temporary measures and will not permanently correct the situation. They must not be placed and forgotten. They require periodic removal, cleaning, reinsertion, and care. Various types of surgery are often recommended to provide permanent correction. These are decisions to be made in consultation with your gynecologist.

Some women find that when they laugh, cough, sneeze, or do anything stressful, including heavy lifting, they lose some urine. This is called stress incontinence. The amount of urine lost varies from a few drops to a puddle. It may be necessary to wear a sanitary pad to prevent soiling clothing and embarrassment. In addition, many women are disturbed by the odor they have because of the constant dribbling of urine. Keeping the bladder empty by frequent urination will minimize the amount of urine lost, and minipads that can be changed frequently will reduce the odor problems. This problem is seen most frequently in women who have had children, but some women who have never been pregnant have this difficulty. It may start well before menopause and get progressively worse with the passage of years. It is due to the relaxation of the tissues around the bladder neck and the inability of the urinary sphincter to tighten appropriately. Hormones are no help here, but Kegel's exercises may be effective. To do them you voluntarily tighten up the muscles you use to avoid urinating. To practice, attempt to stop and start the urine flow at will. Your doctor will tell you how frequently and how often these exercises should be done. Surgery may ultimately be necessary. Even surgery is not 100 percent curative. Since urinary tract infections may cause similar symptoms, medical attention is imperative.

The atrophic changes described above are not confined to the genital areas but they can affect other mucous membranes as well. If your nose is affected, the drying of the mucous membranes may leave you with a constant unpleasant odor. If your eyes are affected, you may find that you are unable to tear and the normal moisture of the eye is lacking. This leads to an unpleasant dryness that can be very discomforting. Oral estrogen therapy will usually aid both these difficulties.

OSTEOPOROSIS

Osteoporosis is the loss of the mineral *calcium* from the bones, and this demineralization causes bones to become porous. As a result, those bones which bear pressure or have muscles pulling on them may collapse. The backbones (vertebrae) are the most often affected and the visible result is the shortened or stooped stature of the aged. In addition, chronic back pain and muscle spasms develop and are persistent. Osteoporosis is a gradual process which affects some women much more than others.

For example, Ms. J. G., now sixty-eight years of age, had remembered herself as being sixty-four inches most of her life. Over the past ten years, though, she has noticed that she is shrinking, and on a recent physical examination was found to measure sixty-two inches. In addition, her posture is stooped, and she can no longer hold herself erect. She has been complaining of chronic, nagging low back pain for years and had never been given a satisfactory explanation for it.

In addition to causing postural problems, loss of calcium also leaves the bones brittle with a tendency to break easily from minor falls. Broken hips from tripping and skidding on icy terrain in the winter are a hazard for older postmenopausal women. Bed rest and immobilization of the broken limb or area only compounds the problem because of the increased demineralization that occurs under these circumstances.

It is difficult to determine when the actual onset of osteoporosis begins. The disease process as described above is usually seen in women who are well past their menopause and into their sixties or seventies, but it does not start then. Probably the demineralization of the bones begins around forty without producing any symptoms. Even after clinical symptoms develop, the diagnosis is not always easily made because of the lack of objective findings. There may be a loss of calcium from the bone, but there is no objective way of measuring this. Blood tests are not useful, and laboratory studies are valueless. The loss of calcium must be extensive before it will show up on an X ray. Obviously, under these conditions, early diagnosis is impossible and the doctor may not be able to find anything wrong. There are many things that may cause low back pain: overexercising, bruises, muscle spasm from heavy lifting, etc. Not every case of back pain is due to osteoporosis. The dilemma for a physician is to determine if back symptoms are early signs of osteoporosis. Exclusion of other reasons for low back pain is generally how the diagnosis is made, but it may take many years to confirm.

Why this calcium loss occurs is truly unknown. Men do not experience it as often as women. Because it appears after menopause the lack of sex steroids and hormones has been blamed. Loss of estrogen in particular has been equated with the onset of osteoporosis. For this reason, women who show marked osteoporotic changes are often put on estrogen replacement therapy in the hope of reversing these changes. As far as we know at this time, replacement therapy with estrogen may slow down the process of demineralization but will not halt it completely. Calcium loss continues to occur. Estrogen is of value only for those women in whom the calcium loss is extensive. In the majority of women, the use of estrogen has not been shown to be beneficial for this problem. Doctors simply do not know how to replace the lost calcium once it is gone. Poor nutrition with inadequate calcium intake may be to blame, and it is a good idea to make sure your diet is adequate in calcium. Improved dietary habits and replacement of calcium will not mean that the bones will become remineralized, but doctors recommend this in the attempt to slow down the process of osteoporosis.

DEPRESSION

Approximately 10 to 30 percent of women who are menopausal will develop emotional disturbances, but these disturbances are not clearly symptoms of menopause. Although frequently attributed to the menopause, depression probably has little to do with the loss of estrogen.

CHANGES IN PHYSIQUE

As the menopause nears and passes, you may note that your body configuration changes. You may find that you have a tendency to gain weight, even to become obese. Acquiring a matronly figure with broader hips and thickened waist may be depressing. In addition, you may note that you lose some tissue from your upper arms. There is an apparent and real redistribution of fat at this time. There is much women can do to minimize these changes.

The increase in weight occurs because women continue to consume as many calories as they did at age twenty. If with increasing age you become more sedentary, you really do not need to eat as much to maintain your weight. The same number of calories coupled with decreased activity leads to an increase in weight. To some extent, the tendency may be cultural. It is interesting to note that obesity in this age group does not exist in China or India.

In addition, lack of exercise will lead to the loss of muscle tone and the appearance of flabbiness. You therefore not only increase your weight but appear very flabby also. Weight and flabbiness may respond to reducing diets and an increase in the amount you exercise.

The breasts go through several changes during the climacteric period. With the advent of anovulatory cycles, your breasts may actually begin to increase somewhat in size as a result of the unopposed estrogen that is present. As the estrogen levels begin to decrease around menopause, your breasts may begin to shrink and become wrinkled and sagging. Hormonal replacement will not restore the firm, round breasts of your youth. Wrinkling of the skin is probably due to the loss of elasticity and a decrease of the tissue beneath your skin caused by the aging process; it is not under hormonal control. Local skin creams or medications taken by mouth are of no value to you if restoration of your skin tone is the anticipated result.

As you go through the menopause and are adjusting to all your bodily changes, you may begin to notice the appearance of some coarse hairs around your chin. In very rare cases, the hair is extensive and may even look like a beard. Growth occurs as a result of the loss of estrogen and the relative dominance of the adrenal hormones which are androgenic in their activity. This problem is relatively easy to solve. If facial hair is annoying or unsightly, it can be bleached or removed by electrolysis or by a facial depilatory. Applying local estrogen creams to your face will not stop the hairs from appearing. Oral estrogen replacement therapy will prevent further hair growth but will not eliminate those hairs already present.

OTHER CHANGES

There are many symptoms that you may experience during your menopause, but it is important to remember that they have probably been bothering you for years—menopause only seems to intensify them. As an example, headaches do not usually accompany menopause, but when they do, they occur more frequently in women who have been prone to this difficulty in the past. Insomnia is another example of a complaint that some women have lived with for years and yet may find intolerable during this period of their life. Insomnia, coupled with sleep disturbed by waking up with a hot flush will cause daytime exhaustion. If you are having this problem, it is not surprising that you then become irritable and short tempered.

Another change many women notice is a change in libido (sex drive). Some women experience an increase in their sex drive, others find no change at all. A few women report that their sex drive has fallen off. If you are someone who has never enjoyed sex, then there is no reason to suspect that things will improve just because you are going through your menopause—unless your dislike of sex is caused by fear of pregnancy. For the most part, those women who have reported diminished libido are usually the same ones who have had sexual problems in the past.

Constipation is a problem of aging that hormonal therapy will not alleviate. In our bowel-conscious society, everyone becomes concerned about the frequency and consistency of their bowel movements. Actually, as part of the aging process, the smooth muscle of the intestinal wall may relax and the intestines may not work as efficiently as they had in the past. You will therefore become more aware of constipation. A change in dietary habits usually helps, and if you increase roughage (green, leafy vegetables) and your fluid intake, you can avoid having to rely on laxatives.

REGULAR CHECKUPS

Because heart disease, high blood pressure, strokes, diabetes, and cancer all become more prevalent among older men and women, I recommend that everyone have a regular annual examination by their physician. These disease processes, if present, may mask or mimic the menopausal or postmenopausal symptoms and may contribute to what seem to be problems of menopause. Early detection and diagnosis of disease processes will enable you to live a longer and healthier life.

It is reassuring to know that most women go through menopause with relatively minor symptoms, if any, and that most of those with more serious problems can get help from their doctors.

3

THE EMOTIONAL ELEMENT

"I'm in the middle of a divorce. I have three children—had three children but one was killed in an accident. I've got to find a way to support myself but I'm not sure how. I've tried selling—I've tried being an automobile saleswoman, but I just can't sell cars. In college I was an art major, and I guess art has been my real love—painting—but I've let it go."

"My wonderful husband has been gone for several years. I'm a widow. I used to have friends but now that I'm all alone they don't invite me any more. I've kept myself up and I think some of these wives who have let themselves go see me as a threat. I keep hoping I'll meet someone. I take vacations. I hope that soon I'll meet my Prince Charming."

Both of these quotes come from women who are undergoing "the change of life." Both women are depressed. Their particular problems typify the emotional disasters women fear as they enter their forties and fifties. And, in addition to fears about real life crises, there are the doubts and anxieties about menopause. "How emotionally difficult is menopause?" "Am I going to become nagging, anxious, depressed?" "Will I go mad?" Questions such as these torment women on the verge of menopause. They are born of myth, of misinformation, and of the particular stresses and strains of our society. To answer them we need to examine the present realities of being a woman, discard the myths, and cope with the actual emotional hazards that exist in our changing world.

In fact, that period of a woman's psychobiological life during which she stops menstruating is potentially stressful; as in adolescence, hormonal changes may cause physical symptoms and, as in adolescence, fear of the bodily changes which occur may provoke emotional reactions. Unlike adolescence, however, the menopause has not been given much attention by sociological, psychological, or medical researchers. Women are left to gather odd bits and pieces of information from dubious or misguided sources: sensational women's magazine articles (a story last year in *The Ladies' Home Journal* revealed that Rosemary Clooney had entered a mental institution at the time of her menopause), gynecologists who never question our society's biased vision of older women as useless relics, or friends and relatives who proclaim that menopause is either an unmitigated nightmare of hot flashes and anxiety or an event with no significance whatsoever. The truth of the matter is that menopause does not provoke madness. The great majority of women experience, at the most, minor episodes of anxiety or depression. Yet, while some women sail through this period of their lives with never a symptom or a tear, it is equally misguided to underestimate the significance of the menopause in a woman's emotional life.

THE STRESS POINTS

The course of our psychobiological development is marked by events of critical significance, and the way we handle these events depends greatly on our self-images as women. The first period (the menarche), the first sexual experience, pregnancy, and the delivery of the first child—all are stress points. Some women approach these experiences with eagerness and wonder, others with dread. Often, the women who have had difficulty with their first periods, who have experienced this sign of womanhood as a loss of freedom or badge of inferiority, are the ones who have the most difficulty with menopause, complaining the most about symptoms and suffering the most from depression and related emotional problems. In a sense, this is a paradox. Having endured the burden of menstruation, these women might be expected to welcome the freedom that the menopause brings. But what they really are expressing is their fear, anger, and disappointment at being women. Other failures in life are rationalized as menopausal problems. The process of menopause is uniquely female and may stir up a whole complex of bitterness and resentment.

Often the causes are very real and can be traced to a society that regards women as second-class citizens. Time and again I have heard accounts of mothers abusing their young daughters because they have begun to menstruate. This abuse may take the form of neglect: girls were not informed by their mothers about menstruation, hence, "I didn't know what a period was"; of denigration: Words like *the curse* are used to label menstruation as bad; or overt hostility. One mother slapped her daughter when the girl announced she was having a period; although this is a custom in some societies, it is nonetheless a "castrating" gesture. Abusive mothers are products of a social system that discriminates against and abuses women, and one hopes that as women gain greater equality and freedom to make choices, the biological events which mark us as female won't carry such a bitter emotional burden. There is no reason why these events should not be greeted with joy.

Women who have had satisfying lives and have not felt hampered by their femaleness will experience the changes of menopause with the same degree of ease with which they have greeted the other major events of their reproductive lives. Think back on your own experiences. If you had a relatively uncomplicated time with your first period, if you were able to adjust to being a new mother—without major postpartum depression—and if your relationships are generally good, including that with your husband, the chances are that you will have few problems with feelings of loss and depression at menopause. Any symptoms you do experience will be milder and less frightening to you than to a woman who has experienced marked difficulty with her other psychobiological stress points. ("Difficulty," of course, does not mean a few period cramps or a few hours of "the blues," problems which almost everyone experiences.) The woman who feels good about the way she has lived her life up until menopause, who has satisfying human relationships, who gets satisfaction from work and pleasure from recreation, who has real and developed interests of her own—apart from home, husband, and children—is not going to have a sudden inexplicable depression at menopause. Those women who do become depressed often have what is referred to as a "depressed life-style": that is, they have always been depressed and menopause only exacerbates an existing condition.

WHAT WE MAY FEAR

It is important to recognize the role that fear plays in the emotional problems of menopause, to face and explore that fear. Almost all of us have feared in some measure loss of attractiveness as we grow older. Menopause is a specific symbol of the passing of time. It marks the end of the reproductive years. Will we continue to be desirable sex partners, and will we be valuable people if we cannot produce children (one of the major values our culture attaches to femaleness)? We fear that hormonal changes will affect our ability to enjoy sex. Such fears are only natural when we stop and consider the emphasis our society puts on youthfulness and beauty and now, increasingly, on sexual performance.

Those fears that are the result of ignorance can be dispelled or greatly reduced when the physiology of menopause is clearly explained and we come to realize that the whole process of ceasing to menstruate is really very gradual. Long before a woman notices that she's having some menstrual irregularity, there has been an extremely slow tapering off of her ovarian function and hormone production. When we stop thinking of menopause as a sudden shutdown, we may find it seems less frightening. We may also find reassurance in the fact that medical treatment is available for specific symptoms of menopause. Once we realize that we are not going to undergo some drastic change, we can stop worrying about menopause in particular and try to focus on our feelings about the general process of aging.

The most basic fear people experience as they grow older is the fear of a loss of control. There are changes that occur in our bodies over which we have absolutely no control. We cannot decide to remain young and fertile forever. Time carries us along willy-nilly and nothing we can do will stop our growing old. Menopause is the stress point that crystallizes this fear. Mothers find that their children are suddenly grown or nearly self-sufficient. Women who are married may find that their husbands are less available, either immersed in work, plagued by their own fears of loss of potency, or out having an affair. Women who are single or divorced face the reality of remaining partnerless for the remainder of their lives. This is the bleak side of these middle years, a set of problems many women have never fantasized or foreseen. Those women who were good wives and mothers but never did anything outside the home often find their sense of importance stripped away. They may feel that the whole worth of their lives is called into question and that there is very little they can do—or even could have done—to prevent what seems to be a breakdown of the home and family they strove to create and maintain. Of course, there are things they *can* do, as will be discussed later, but the point is that it is from these fears that the emotional problems of menopause arise. And these fears and problems are exacerbated by changes at this time in a woman's life situation and by society's very negative image of "the older woman."

HOW SOCIETY TAKES ITS TOLL

How do we see ourselves as women? Who are our models? And what do we expect we must do to be successful? These are some of the questions women in general are asking themselves. The answers we give are as often determined by images and ideas which are external to us, which are imposed on us by our world, as they are determined by inner perceptions. In the press, in women's magazines, in men's magazines, in movies, and on television women seem to exist only visually. Newspaper articles characterize women by age and hair color—"an attractive thirty-two-year-old brunette" describes a woman lawyer, though her male counterpart would never be described as a handsome thirty-two-year-old blond. It hardly seems necessary at this point to paint the whole grim media picture, and there are signs of change here, but women (and men) have spent too many years immersed in propaganda to be able to escape its effects easily. Young women exist too often as faces and bodies that sell cigarettes or perfume, that model clothes, that offer sex without strings attached, that decorate the arms of successful and enterprising men.

When we come to the middle-aged woman, we find a less alluring image. Now she is the nagging older wife or mother-in-law or the nosy neighbor. What is even more disturbing, however, is the negative image of the older woman in the advertising aimed at those doctors who must help and advise her. One recent ad for a hormone replacement drug, for example, shows a worried older woman (presumably suffering from symptoms of menopause) saying, "I know what happened to my mother. It wasn't just how she looked. There was her back stiff and bent, bladder trouble—I dreaded it." Bladder trouble and bent backs are not direct results of ovarian deficiency, and it is this kind of advertising that creates negative expectations in the gynecologists who are the main treatment resources for women undergoing menopausal distress. How many movies can you think of where the heroine is a vital, attractive, interesting middle-aged woman? How many television programs portray a middle-aged woman in a positive way?

The effects of these constant negative images on the individual should not be taken lightly. The beleaguered middle-aged woman, portrayed effectively by Elizabeth Taylor in the movie *Ash Wednesday*, tries to eradicate the dreaded signs of age in order to win back her husband, who has left her for a younger woman. In a desperate attempt to compete with youthful attractiveness, she undergoes plastic surgery. In real life, a patient of mine in the same situation tried the same thing. Unfortunately the surgery went badly, and she looked worse than before. (All surgery has its risks, and plastic surgery is no exception.) Sometimes, no matter how good the result, the woman will be gravely disappointed, because her *real* expectation is that surgery will change her life, not just her appearance. My patient was an attractive, stylish physician was was remarkably youthful looking. Her decision was based not on a realistic appraisal of her looks but on the desperate hope of becoming young, beautiful, and once again desirable to her husband. If she were able to accept herself as an attractive middle-aged woman, she might have questioned her husband's motivation, and put the blame on their bad relationship, or *his* lack of judgment in leaving, rather than on *her* own face, her surface. Or she might instead have looked *within* herself to find causes for the deterioration of her marriage.

Women who pursue the "youth cult" find it requires a kind of sacrificial torture. Doctors who can tighten thighs, carve up breasts and buttocks, and restructure chins are in demand. Although the youth cult also oppresses men, women are the primary victims and will continue to be until changes in our society create a new climate—one in

THE EMOTIONAL ELEMENT

which individual character and accomplishment are the valuable things about people, one in which the beautiful people are those with beautiful souls—and in this case they are bound to be physically attractive as well.

There are hopeful signs in some of the effects of the women's movement: more novels by women which explore what it means to be female in America, more movies by women film-makers which portray women of accomplishment, and a greater reluctance in young women today to accept restrictions on their goals or freedom simply because of their sex. Finally, there are certain women, busy and self-confident, who are able to ignore the media puffery of surface glamor. They go about the lives they have created with a strong sense of self. And the stress of menopause is for them simply a normal change to be accepted for whatever problems or benefits it might bring. In truth, the symptoms of the actual physical menopause do not have to be accompanied by any psychological feelings whatsoever beyond a brief recognition that the event punctuates the end of reproductive life and heralds the beginning of a new phase—often one of real freedom, serenity, and satisfaction.

WHEN PROBLEMS OCCUR

Some women *do* have emotional problems at menopause, for the reasons explored in the preceding pages. And these are legitimate reasons. By far the most common emotional problem is depression. Many women experience mild depression at the time of menopause, occasional bouts of the blues which may serve a protective function at a time when there is a need for a regrouping of psychic forces. Of course, some serious depressions may occur.

What are the signs of depression? One way to describe this condition is to point out that for the depressed person time is slowed down. She can't move as quickly. Speech is slowed down. Changes in basic life rhythms are another sign. Depression can cause loss of appetite or a sudden need to eat all the time, insomnia or a need to sleep long hours. Waking at an increasingly earlier hour is a classic sign of depression. Depressed people are tearful and engage in self-accusations: "I'm no good" or "I wasn't a good mother" or "Nobody loves me" are typical sentiments of depression. Freud has pointed out that these accusations against the self are in reality accusations of others, i.e., "*You* don't love me." At the stress point of menopause, fear of loss of love or of attractiveness provokes anger, which is then directed against the self. Menopause itself does not "cause" depression, mild or serious, but it can be the occasion for the intensification of preexisting depression because there is a noticeable change to fix on.

Perhaps one of the most typical dilemmas faced by women at the time of menopause was given concrete imagery in the following dream of a depressed patient of mine. The problem presented in this dream lies at the heart of many emotional problems that women struggle with at this period of their lives.

In her dream the woman goes to a hotel remembered from her past and finds it changed. It is the same, yet different. When she asks for a room she is refused one, and "when I want to dine in the hotel restaurant they don't seem to want me there. I find myself standing in the lobby, and the floor begins to shake. Suddenly, I am simultaneously lying on the floor inside, clinging to something, and yet seeing outside the hotel, where to one side there is a huge excavation where a huge modern building is to be put up. I realize that the little old hotel is collapsing and falling into the excavation. I try to keep holding on and I think, 'Would I still be able to—if I give up clinging on here—will I still be able to get out the front door and be saved?' At this point I wake up."

This patient woke up in a state of great anxiety, not knowing whether she could have been saved or not. As I interpret the dream, the hotel was both new and old, which suggests her early life and what she had now become. She was in the hotel, and there was something in herself and/or in her life with which she was unfamiliar. Somehow or other she wasn't welcome in the hotel. You might say that she felt life would not accept her and would not feed her. And in the image of a building collapsing she saw herself and wondered how she could save herself: by clinging to the new/old building she saw as herself or trying to escape out the door, which seemed an empty escape.

This woman, facing menopause, faces a new stage in her development. With the loss of reproductive ability comes a new freedom: The childbearing, child-raising years are over and she has—statistically —a quarter of a century ahead. How will she use these years? She is both new and old. Fearful as the new may seem, it has the potential to be gratifying.

MENOPAUSE FOR THE WOMAN ALONE

If you are divorced, about to be divorced, widowed, or single, and feeling unhappy or anxious or depressed about your singlehood, the menopause may loom large. What will the older years offer? Can life be satisfactory at this point. Will there be compensations? Divorce is a stressful event; so is the death of a husband. Lack of money and the insecurity of not having another person to share your life may cause extreme anxiety, but this need not be the case. Some women find these years to be the most productive and exciting ones yet; this is a time to become reacquainted with yourself, to explore new relationships, or to redevelop old ones long ignored.

One patient of mine, an art lover but timid about her ability, had not painted seriously for many years. Although I encouraged her to use some of her free time to paint, she seemed unable to do it. Then a former friend called her up to say that he was in town, to see a museum exhibit—would she come along? They went to dinner and he gave her a very practical idea: Why not, he suggested, work in the art world, using her excellent organizational skills? She was delighted with her evening and became interested enough to begin painting again. She also followed up on his suggestion and is now a business manager of a small gallery. Now that she is busy and active, she's happier with herself and, incidentally, has increased her chances of meeting men. It took this woman time to change her life, but she did it.

WHERE ARE THE MEN OF YESTERYEAR?

As the song says, a good man is hard to find. For the woman who is interested in having more than a casual relationship, finding an interesting, mature, attractive man can pose a knotty problem. It may seem that all the men you know are either married and taken, married and interested in a secret affair, or footloose and on the prowl for younger women. Some women enjoy brief or casual sex; they are either very busy with other parts of their lives or just not interested in living with a man. Others, believing in monogamous committed relationships, may find the one-night stand an excruciating affront to their sense of self-worth. Which group are you in? It is important to be truly honest with yourself about this question. Agreeing to have sex with a man when you have serious expectations that this will lead to love and marriage lets you in for an emotional beating. If you can enjoy the encounter for what it is worth and remain very open in what you expect it will lead to, then go ahead. But if you believe that sex is wrong or meaningless unless it occurs within the context of a committed relationship, you must weigh the emotional consequences to your own sense of self-esteem.

What is important if you are in this situation is to open up your life to as many possibilities as you can: a rewarding job, a serious interest—whether it is a return to a long-neglected early interest, or a new one, like photography, fund-raising for a charity, or a new friendship. You should have many open lines to the larger world and out of this widening circle of acquaintances may come opportunities to meet the kind of men you enjoy, who will in turn appreciate *you*.

LIVING WELL ALONE, OR NOT SO ALONE

Learning to live well and happily by yourself is an enormous challenge. If you've been single for many years, you know the problems and you've had to cope with them. If, however, you're recently divorced or widowed at the time of your menopause, you have to cope with fear of loneliness at a stressful time, when you may mistrust your ability to make a new life. The solution to your living situation is very much a question of your own needs. If you can adjust to new people, having an apartment- or house-mate is often practical and pleasant. You can share expenses and have the security of knowing that there's someone around should problems arise. People are finding all sorts of ways to share their lives with others. Maybe you can give a room to a college student. If you have energy and love children you might consider the possibility of adopting an older child or providing foster care. (State laws are increasingly flexible on the issue of who may adopt.) Withdrawing into your own shell is the danger at this point. One antidote is to find a group of people in your situation to talk things over with. You will be surprised how many "rap groups" filled with interesting people are being formed at YWCAs, women's centers, churches, temples, and community centers. And if there isn't one, why not begin one? You know there is a need.

AS THE TWIG IS BENT

One point I make to mothers, especially mothers of daughters, is that the way they handle the fears and tensions of the menopausal period will set an example to their children. It is not a question of "being brave for the sake of the children" but a realization that there are still important things you may teach by example. If you are clinging, demanding, and complaining, you are teaching your child that this is what menopause does to a woman. Does it? Another important lesson that a menopausal mother may teach, either badly or well, is the lesson of preparation. A woman who has neglected herself, her mind, and her interests and who has lost her identity in the housewife/mother role has a harder time in creating a new life than does the woman who has continued to work, has maintained an interest in her appearance and in the broader world, or who has pursued some serious interest apart from the daily (and yes, demanding) routine of housework and child care. A woman who has not prepared herself in her youth for more than this role is in for a tough time. And this is a lesson that high school- and college-age daughters would do well to learn early. If you're the mother of one, you can give valuable support to her ambitions and goals in the area of career and self-development.

DO YOU NEED PSYCHOTHERAPY?

How do you know if you could benefit from therapy? How do you know if you need it? This is obviously a tricky area; our profession holds that we could all probably benefit from some sort of help. And yet, sometimes a talk with a close friend may be all some people need to get them through a rough spot in their lives. If you feel seriously depressed and the depression gets worse or fails to lighten, if you carry a burden of fears which prevent you from living an active normal life, if you feel helpless to change your situation, then you may need professional help in working out your problems and uncovering new solutions to what you consider a hopeless state of affairs. Keep in mind that therapy is work and requires the active, intelligent cooperation of the patient for real success. You must be willing to take a look at yourself if you want to make progress and achieve change.

WHAT KIND OF THERAPY?

The kind of treatment I have found most helpful is what therapists call "total push." This approach uses every tool at hand to alleviate the depression and other symptoms and to direct the patient back on the road to an active, interesting life. Antidepressant drugs which are *carefully* prescribed can be very helpful. The goal of the therapist is to mobilize the patient to take an active interest in her destiny rather than drift passively through life. Sometimes the first steps are very small ones. For a woman who's given up entertaining friends, it may mean inviting an old friend over for coffee or supper. The effort of entertaining draws her back into contact with people, and she sends out signals by her action: "Look, I'm trying to stay in touch. Why don't you?" It is doing something *active* for herself, rather than just passively drifting. For some women, a woman therapist who draws on a personal understanding of what it is to lead a woman's life can be extremely helpful, and is potentially more empathetic. For other women, especially those who have always looked to men for guidance, a woman therapist will not represent enough authority to be useful.

HOW TO FIND A THERAPIST

It can be difficult to choose a therapist. One way to approach the problem is to consult your family physician or internist, who can do a thorough medical evaluation to rule out the possibility of an organic problem and can then refer you to an appropriate therapist. Hospitals that have mental health programs are a good source for referrals, as are community mental health programs and other community service organizations such as those sponsored by various religious groups. If your income falls below a certain limit, you may be able to use these services; if not, they can usually offer you an evaluation plus referrals to psychiatrists, licensed psychologists, and certified social workers, depending on your emotional needs and financial resources.

HOW TO KNOW IF YOU HAVE CHOSEN THE "RIGHT" THERAPIST

The best way to judge the effectiveness of your therapist is through your own instinctive reaction. You need to ask yourself these questions: Is this person really sympathetic to *my* problems? Is this person really concerned about me? If you feel ill at ease with your therapist and have a sense that you are not making progress, you need to discuss it openly in one of your sessions, and if you're not satisfied with his or her answers, you need to consider the possibility that you ought to change. If you have changed therapists several times with no better reaction, though, you may have to consider whether or not the problem lies within yourself. You must follow your best judgment in this. Good professional qualifications are a guide, but they are not the *only* basis for a decision.

WHAT TO DO IF YOU ARE TROUBLED AND CAN'T OR WON'T SEEK PROFESSIONAL HELP

Therapy speeds recovery from depression and other emotional problems; yet, there are other ways to help yourself if you're unable to get counseling. Basically, it's the *desire* to change and the search for sources of emotional strength that lead to recovery. You may uncover sources of help among friends and relatives that will get you through this time of readjustment. A sympathetic husband, for example, can be a source of comfort and reassurance to a wife who is undergoing emotional stress. A husband cannot play therapist but he and his wife, by sharing feelings, can gain greater closeness during a difficult time.

CAN YOU TALK TO YOUR CHILDREN?

There are ways of creating better communications with your children that can help you to increase your (and their) pleasure in talking together and being together. If you've fallen into the trap of being a know-it-all parent, you've cut yourself off from a very rich area of closeness and sharing. Take some time to wonder who your children really are, what they think, what they dream. Rather than telling them what's best for them, why not ask for their opinion on subjects you're concerned about, whether it's selecting the right color for a carpet or predicting the future of Western civilization? Instead of being automatically critical of your children, stop and explore their points of view, their reasons for making the choices they do. I have two grown children, both doctors, and I've always looked forward to sharing knowledge with them and getting their reactions to things I was reading and thinking. I always felt that my daughter particularly had the edge on *me*, in intellectual brilliance and matters of taste. Even though she lives quite far away, we share our experiences in letters and look forward to discussing our work when we get together. My children and I can talk together as equals on a professional level, something that is unusual; but there really are endless ways to communicate as equals if you give up the role of parent as stern judge of all behavior. So this can be a time of drawing closer together through a renewed appreciation of mutual interests and abilities.

REVIVING FRIENDSHIPS

In addition to trying to open up new lines of communication with husband and children, you might take time to consider the state of your friendships. One patient of mine was trying to cope with a depression and one of the possibilities we explored was the reestablishing of friendships she'd let dwindle away. She'd neglected her friends. In her preoccupation with her own problems, she'd retreated from the world. So she set about calling and writing people she knew and liked. Some were indifferent, but others were thrilled to hear from her and as happy to revive the friendship as she. Cooking a special dinner for friends, going to the theater, going on a trip—there are so many possibilities. And most of all, the busier you are, the less time there will be for noticing any discomforts you may feel.

THE VIRTUES OF SELF-INDULGENCE

On the other side of the coin, perhaps the most important person to open up lines of communication with is yourself. This is a time when you should be exploring your own wants and needs. Now that you've spent a number of years raising a family or working—or both— you deserve to focus on things that you want and have put off doing.

One woman who'd raised four active children in a no-frills kind of decor had always had a passion for fragile, breakable, pretty things; now she was able to buy and decorate her home with the frail teacups and blown-glass objects she'd always had to resist before. A small luxury, hardly a major change in outlook or goals, but still, having those things made her feel good. Another woman had always loved nice clothes but in the effort to raise and educate her children had felt she couldn't afford more than the most basic suits and raincoats. She now takes great pleasure in buying things she doesn't absolutely *have* to have. For some women, reading for pleasure had to be put off while growing children made demands on time and attention; now they are able to do the reading they dreamed of doing. A word of caution here: It is not easy to get back to long-abandoned interests, especially if they call for a certain amount of effort, but with a little persistence, it can be accomplished.

INTELLECTUAL GROWTH

You reach the end of physical growth in your early twenties, but there need be no limit to your intellectual development. Rather than complain that your husband is buried in the newspaper, why not buy another copy and immerse yourself? There is a larger world beyond home and family, and it has been one of the ongoing struggles of the feminist movement to allow women to engage in that larger world and to make their share of decisions in it. Increasingly, colleges and universities have been opening their doors to the older people who are returning to continue (or make up for a lack of) their education. Some institutions have special programs for mature women. Whether you are trying for a degree or taking courses in specific areas of interest, this is a good time to reexplore the life of the mind.

REALISTIC EXPECTATIONS

As you set out to create a basis for this next stage of your life, you need to make realistic decisions. The second quote at the beginning of this chapter was from a woman who was determined to wait for her Prince Charming, and I suspect that she is waiting still. Hers is not a realistic expectation. If you are interested in meeting and attracting men, make yourself as attractive as possible and then go out into the world to meet *them*. If you want to work, assess your skills (and you may have more than you think), and then look for work in an area in which you have practical ability. You may not become an Olympic track star, but perhaps you can run a sports program for children. You may not play first violin in the orchestra, but perhaps you have public relations ability and can work to promote the orchestra. It is unrealistic to be overly pessimistic, depressed, and unable to appreciate who you are. It is also unrealistic to demand all or nothing. Maybe you haven't met Prince Charming, but perhaps you can have an encounter at a museum or a good conversation at a dinner party with an interesting man. It's a start.

THE HEALTHY MENOPAUSAL WOMAN

Having discussed many of the problems that beset the woman facing and entering upon the menopausal period, we now must ask: What is a successful menopause? How does the emotionally healthy woman experience it? First, she does not necessarily have doubts and fears about loss of sexual attractiveness at this time. If she does, she understands these fears are exacerbated by our youth-oriented culture. But if she has had a reasonably happy and satisfactory sex and love life, she values herself; her sense of self-worth keeps her from becoming a victim of each new wrinkle or gray hair. She enjoys close relationships with friends, with her husband, with her children. If unmarried, she may share many aspects of life with a lover. She has strong interests beyond the home, and she pursues those interests. She welcomes the freedom to do new things that her children's independence gives her. Rather than blaming life for her unhappiness, she goes out to discover what else it has to offer.

4

ESTROGEN: WHAT TO DO UNTIL THE RESULTS ARE IN

THE BIG QUESTION

Since 1931, when the first woman patient received the first dose of the newly isolated female hormone *estrogen*, millions of women have received estrogen therapy for a variety of reasons: for birth control, menstrual problems, failure of ovaries to develop, and, of course, for relief of the symptoms of menopause. Estrogen has proven itself very effective in some of its uses, dubious in others. And now, in the mid-1970s, we are beginning to learn more about its long-term effects. There are risks involved in its use, and perhaps because of the fervor with which some physicians promoted it as a fountain of youth, there is now public anxiety and a sense of betrayal. Estrogen[1], that panacea that promised to prevent everything from wrinkles to depression, is now associated with a possible increase in risk from endometrial cancer.

For women approaching menopause or experiencing symptoms of menopause, whether or not to take estrogen is a very big, very real question—and one which is difficult to answer in the present climate of anxiety. To understand how such controversy has arisen over a chemical which our own glands produce, with which we live in harmony for years, and which determines our very femaleness, we need to distinguish between the estrogen produced by our own bodies to

---

1. Only estrogen replacement therapy is being discussed here; as we go to press, birth control pills are considered *free* of increased risk of endometrial cancer.

regulate a variety of normal functions and the estrogen (whether natural or synthetic) that we use as a drug to relieve symptoms or correct malfunctions.

DISCOVERY OF THE "FEMALE PRINCIPLE"

Long before anyone knew that such things as hormones existed, people recognized that there was a relationship between certain glands and sexual development. For example, centuries ago young males were castrated in order to provide eunuchs to guard the sultans' harems or supply church choirs with the high pure voices of the *castrati*, those perpetual boy sopranos. Loss of testicles meant loss of male characteristics. Although the Greeks and Romans realized that the ovaries were responsible in some undefined way for the development and maintenance of a woman's reproductive function, it was not until the middle of the nineteenth century that research began on the substances called hormones: a number of different chemicals produced in minute quantities by specialized glands, each carried by the blood stream to a certain part of the body which it regulates. We know today that there are three basic sex hormones produced by women: estrogen, progesterone, and androgen. All three of these hormones working together are necessary for normal sexual development and the regulation of reproduction and menstruation. It is estrogen, however, the most potent and the source of controversy, that is the focus of attention in this chapter.

As was the case with most other hormones, evidence for the existence of estrogen came from observing what happened to subjects (animal and human) who had both ovaries removed. In 1900, a Viennese gynecologist, Dr. Emil Knauer, found that doing ovarian transplants prevented the symptoms associated with loss of ovaries. Scientists searched for the "female principle" and eventually isolated the substance that had such profound effects. Today we know a good deal more about its intricate formation and functioning. We can, for example, chart the long, complex, interlocking series of steps that must occur for the formation and utilization of hormones. Several parts of the brain as well as a number of glands such as the thyroid, parathyroid, pancreas, and adrenals are involved. Much research, however, remains to be done before these processes are thoroughly understood.

THE DECISIVE ROLE OF ESTROGEN

Before examining the pluses or minuses of estrogen replacement therapy, it is important to see the way this hormone functions in normal sexual development, of which menopause is, after all, simply the final stage.

The sex of an infant is genetically determined. Two X chromosomes spell female; an XY combination, male. But at first, the developing fetus is undifferentiated. In fact, for the first six weeks of life, boy is indistinguishable from girl. It is the play of specific sex hormones upon the genetic matrix that determines the ultimate male or female appearance of the tiny embryo.

Until birth, there is an abundant supply of estrogen and progesterone furnished by the mother. Often both male and female newborns show signs of breast development, and sometimes milk (called "witch's milk" by the superstitious) actually leaks from their breasts. Several days after delivery, newborn girls may experience a small amount of vaginal bleeding—really a kind of withdrawal bleeding as the maternal estrogen disappears, causing the lining of the baby's uterus to break down. Until they approach puberty, girls produce very little estrogen.

ESTROGEN AND PUBERTY

Estrogen plays the major role in creating a mature woman capable of reproducing her kind.

Just prior to puberty, in response to chemical signals from the brain, the ovaries enlarge and begin to produce the estrogen that is responsible for the major changes of puberty. Estrogen acts on the breasts by causing the area around the nipple to darken and by stimulating the growth of duct tissue. Estrogen is responsible for feminine fat distribution—the typical curves of breast and hips. Estrogen causes the internal reproductive organs to grow. The cervix enlarges. The body of the uterus, the *fundus*, not only enlarges but becomes capable of the striking growth that will be necessary for pregnancy. The blood vessels of the lining of the uterus, the *endometrium*, enlarge and the increased blood supply stimulates the endometrium to grow thicker. The Fallopian tubes grow and, under the influence of estrogen, become able to relax and contract, the motion that will push the egg downward to where fertilization occurs. The vagina is very responsive to estrogen. In the young girl just prior to puberty, the lining of the vagina is very thin, one cell deep; but under the stimulation of estrogen, the lining thickens and both the vagina and the external genitalia, the *labia*, undergo considerable growth. The culmination of this whole sequence of events is the *menarche*, the first menstrual period.

Puberty, like menopause, is a time of physical change and stress. During puberty, the body is flooded with unaccustomed hormones; during the menopausal period the hormones to which the body has acclimated itself are withdrawn, and a new balance must be found. Ironically, in this era of overpopulation, the years between these two events, our reproductive years, are growing longer. The age at which menarche occurs has decreased by roughly four months every ten years since 1800, and there has been a corresponding increase in the age of women at the time of menopause. The reason for this change is unclear, although early evidence points to better nutrition.

Estrogen, in addition to stimulating the development of the female reproductive organs, has other widespread effects on the body as a whole. For example, it increases the water content and thickness of the skin and causes the open growth centers of the bones to close at the end of puberty.

In animals, estrogen causes the "estrus behavior" (the cat in heat, for example), which nature has designed to lead to pregnancy. In human beings sexual behavior is far more complex and harder to explain as simply the result of a particular hormone.

THE OTHER SEX HORMONES

Estrogen does not exert its effects alone. It depends, first of all, upon the biologic responsiveness of the various female organs to stimulation and, second, upon the presence of other hormones, particularly progesterone and androgen. Both estrogen and progesterone are produced by the ovaries in cyclic fashion in response to stimulation from the central nervous system. Androgen, sometimes thought of as exclusively a male hormone, is produced by the adrenal cortex. A normal woman produces about 5 percent of the amount of androgen produced by the normal man. Research indicates that androgen in women is to some extent responsible for growth and for the normal distribution of pubic and underarm hair. (Too much androgen, of course, causes masculinization.)

MEASURING ESTROGEN LEVELS

Researchers have learned how to measure estrogen levels by observing the cyclic changes in every part of a woman's reproductive system during her menstrual cycle. These observations have led to a number of useful tests that can be conducted in the office when a doctor wants to study the hormone levels of a menopausal patient. It is now possible to take samples of tissues, cells, or secretions at different phases of the cycle and learn something about the hormonal status of the donor. For example, one type of test is based on the series of changes that the endometrium undergoes in response to both estrogen and progesterone. By examining a bit of endometrial tissue under the microscope, a pathologist gains excellent information about hormone production and whether or not ovulation is occurring.

A second type of test uses the changes that occur in the cervical secretions during an ovulatory cycle as a basis for chemical and laboratory studies of hormone levels. During each menstrual month, a woman's cervix normally secretes mucus. Early in the menstrual cycle, when estrogen levels are low, there is very little cervical mucus, and what there is has a characteristic thick, gray appearance. It has sometimes been labeled "hostile" mucus because it is virtually impossible for sperm to penetrate. Toward the midpoint of the cycle, when estrogen levels are high, the flow of mucus from the cervix increases and changes. It becomes thin, clear, watery, and receptive to the passage of sperm at the time that the egg becomes ready for fertilization. At midcycle, when there is unopposed estrogen (estrogen is the only hormone present), a phenomenon occurs called *spinnbarkeit*. Cervical secretions smeared on a slide show a characteristic ferning pattern. After this midpoint, the second hormone of the menstrual cycle, *progesterone*, comes into play, and once again the mucus thickens and becomes hostile to sperm.

Knowledge of these changes in women who are menstruating becomes important to physicians evaluating postmenopausal patients who are receiving estrogen and complain of discharge. Women using estrogen preparations may notice the watery discharge characteristic of high estrogen levels and, if it is profuse, may worry that they have developed a vaginal infection. This particular response to estrogen therapy is greatly variable. Some women notice no increase in discharge; for some it is so copious and annoying that therapy must be stopped.

A third type of test, again based on observation of changes in the menstrual cycle, is an examination of cells taken from the vaginal lining. Using a special stain and a microscope, we can determine the stage of the menstrual cycle of the individual from whom the cells have been taken. Toward the beginning and at the end of the cycle, the cells are small, wrinkled, and stain blue. At midcycle, they become large, flat, and stain pink. This is a simple test which will show the type of hormone present and, to some extent, the amount. In a woman with symptoms of menopause this cell maturation test, as it is called, gives some idea of whether or not her symptoms are related to estrogen deficiency—a state revealed by the predominance of small, wrinkled blue cells.

These tests are by no means 100 percent accurate. There are many factors which can influence the result, such as other drugs a woman is taking or a case of vaginitis. There are other more complicated and expensive laboratory tests on samples of blood and urine, which have a somewhat higher degree of accuracy.

ESTROGEN PRODUCTION AT MENOPAUSE AND EVEN BEYOND

Very gradually, our estrogen production slows down. Often in our early forties we may notice changes in our periods due to fluctuating hormone levels because ovulation no longer occurs every month. Somewhere between forty-five and fifty-five (the average age range for menopause) the amount of estrogen our ovaris produce begins to dip below the level necessary to maintain menstruation. For a period of from one to five years, there are missed or irregular periods, heavy bleeding, and/or slight bleeding between periods. Usually, these changes are due to varying levels of estrogen. Although its exact mechanism is uknown, the hot flush is also related to the lack of estrogen; we are sure that this is basically a physical symptom since it is almost always relieved by the administration of estrogen. Other symptoms such as dizziness, headaches, fatigue, and depression may or may not be related to estrogen deprivation. Eventually, after the menopause is complete and the body has adjusted, these symptoms disappear.

Some women experience no symptoms during this time; they just stop menstruating. Others experience one or more symptoms. Even when menopause is over, our adrenal glands continue to manufacture some estrogen. Possibly, women who remain free of symptoms have more active adrenals. There is as yet no accurate way of determining the relation of estrogen levels to all of these symptoms.

In the past three and a half decades increasing numbers of women, wishing to prevent aging, have taken estrogen for various lengths of time, at different dose levels, and in different chemical forms. Some women have had combination therapy of estrogen plus progesterone, or estrogen plus progesterone plus androgen. Originally, the benefits of estrogen replacement therapy seemed obvious, but now the problem of risks has come to the fore. What are those risks and are they so serious that no one should take estrogen? Or are there some women for whom estrogen is necessary and desirable?

HOW WE STUDY THE SIDE EFFECTS OF DRUGS

There is considerable confusion at the present time as to the side effects of estrogen when these hormones are given to menopausal women. Several studies have come out suggesting an apparent association between estrogen therapy and the development of malignancy of the lining of the uterus, and certain vascular complications. More studies are sure to appear. What women need in this era of uncertainty is an understanding of what the studies mean, how they are done, and what constitutes a valid result.

Prospective Studies

To carry out a prospective study, a researcher assembles two groups of patients: One group receives the drug being studied, the other, the *control* group, does not. Both groups are carefully followed to see what happens. In a well-designed prospective study both groups are carefully matched to make sure that they are as alike as possible in age, sex, health, income, and locale—for the researcher wants the only difference between the two groups to be the fact that one is receiving the drug. In the best of these studies, the *double-blind* study, placebos are given to the control group. Everyone gets a pill and no one knows which is the real thing. The researchers who evaluate the results do not know either; they simply assemble and quantify the facts. Not until all the results are in are these facts correlated with the taking of the drug. This is the most objective type of study scientists have been able to devise and it also poses the knottiest ethical problems. All participants in the study must be informed that they may be receiving a drug with possible complications. If it is a potentially valuable new drug, is it being "withheld" from the control group? If it appears to also have side effects, is it being tested on human "victims"? Although it is never possible to predict the full range of effects of a given drug on human beings until many people have taken it, because of FDA regulations this kind of drug testing has become increasingly difficult to do. Usually, rats, hamsters, monkeys, and baboons—the laboratory animals most similar to human beings—are studied and the results are then used to predict the possible side effects in human beings. Since none of these animals is exactly like us, it isn't always possible to know whether or not the information is completely valid.

Retrospective Studies

Another way to gather information on the possible side effects of a drug is to look back at people who have taken it to see what has happened to them. There are two ways of doing this: (1) A group of people who have inadvertently been exposed to a particular substance (workers in a chemical factory, for example) are examined and followed for possible side effects, or (2) a group that has been exposed to a substance or treated with a drug is matched with a control group that has not. In the second example the more factors that are matched in both groups, the more valid the study.

EVALUATING THE RISKS

At the present time, physicians are concerned about a number of conditions (all in the process of being studied) that may be related to the use of estrogen. The first of these is endometrial carcinoma, a cancer of the lining (endometrium) of the uterus. Several reports have been published suggesting that there is a five times higher rate of this malignancy in women who take estrogen than in women who do not. After these studies were presented to the Food and Drug Administration, a bulletin was sent to physicians pointing out the increased risk and suggesting that estrogen be used only when medically indicated, and then only in the lowest dose required to control symptoms. It was further suggested that treatment be discontinued as soon as feasible. Expressing a need for further data to clarify the relationship between the risk of endometrial cancer and factors such as drug dosage, duration of treatment, and cyclical administration, the FDA's Obstetric and Gynecology Advisory Committee concluded that "the studies provided strong evidence that postmenopausal estrogen therapy increases the risk of endometrial cancer." The report in the FDA Drug Bulletin (February–March, 1976) points out that cancer of the endometrium has in the past been rare—one case a year per thousand in postmenopausal women. The annual incidence among estrogen-users, however appears to be four to eight cases per thousand annually. The report continues:

> The usefulness of estrogens in treating certain symptoms of the menopause, especially vasomotor symptoms [hot flashes], is well established. In most women undergoing menopause, however, if psychosomatic symptoms and anxiety predominate, these can often be managed with reassurance and, if necessary, with anti-anxiety medications. If vasomotor symptoms occur they usually need to be treated only for a period of months, rarely for longer than one year. Estrogens are obviously used to a far greater extent and for a far longer time, however, than can be accounted for by the incidence or duration of acute menopausal symptoms. National prescription surveys reveal that annual use of orally administered estrogen is 6 million patient-years and that most of this use is in post-menopausal women. Since less than half of the approximately 1.5 million women who enter the menopause in a single year visit a physician with menopausal complaints and since only a portion of these have major vasomotor symptoms, estrogen use appears to exceed by far that required for short-term management of the menopausal syndrome.

There is obviously an increased risk of endometrial cancer for estrogen users. Is it a great enough risk to rule out the use of estrogen entirely?

RISK VERSUS BENEFIT

That any drug powerful enough to produce a desired effect may, in addition, produce undesired effects in a certain number of patients is a daily reality of modern medicine. One major objective of drug research is to determine the nature and the frequency of any adverse side effects and then to balance these against the known benefits of the particular drug: the *risk versus benefit ratio*. This knowledge allows the physician and his or her patient to make an informed decision as to whether treatment with a particular drug is worth the risks in a particular instance. When a drug is being used for a non-life-threatening situation, the risk associated with its use must be relatively small. When a drug is being given to save a life, the risks may be considerably greater.

There is another concept which physicians use to evaluate the patient's need for a particular drug and that is the quality of the patient's life with or without it. A patient suffering extreme (but not life-threatening) discomfort may be given a drug with certain risks. Such patients must be carefully followed by their physicians to make sure that the drug has no untoward consequences. Estrogen is just such a powerful drug, and when it is prescribed for hot flashes it is being used in a non-life-threatening situation.

Since many millions of women in this country have taken or are currently taking estrogen to alleviate menopausal symptoms it is important to determine whether the risk of endometrial cancer rules out its use for this purpose. In addition, other studies are attempting to determine whether estrogen is related to an increase in breast tumors, whether estrogen users are at greater risk from certain vascular problems, such as thrombophlebitis, myocardial infarction, cerebral thrombosis, and hypertension. At present, it appears that the incidence of each of these with the use of estrogen is quite low. The frequency rises only when other factors are present: smoking, obesity, high blood pressure, or a family history of these diseases. Estrogen also produces metabolic changes in nitrogen balance, lipid and carbohydrate metabolism, and liver function, which may or may not be significant. By and large, when estrogen therapy is discontinued, these changes disappear, usually quite promptly.

THE STUDIES ARE STILL INCONCLUSIVE

We are now in the midst of a great cancer scare; some of our concern is valid, some is perhaps caused by the overreaction of the media. Rarely is the risk versus benefit ratio discussed in the usual newspaper account of a newly suspected cause of cancer. And while studies may point to an increase in cancer, the studies themselves are sometimes faulty or inconclusive. The 1974 data on overall incidence of cancer in the United States show that endometrial cancer is still an uncommon cause of death for women—2,252 deaths listed in that year, accounting for only 1.38 percent of all female deaths from cancer.

MANY FACTORS

On December 15, 1975, an article, "The Cancer Statistics," was published in *Newsweek* suggesting that in the first six months of that year the death rate from endometrial cancer had shot up to five times its previous rate. But, several months later, on careful evaluation of the data, the National Center for Health Statistics noted that there was also an influenza epidemic. It was then suggested that perhaps the increase in the cancer death rate was due to the fact that patients already seriously ill with cancer died when they contracted influenza. There was a second report of increased endometrial cancer deaths in the San Francisco Bay area. It is a mistake, however, to assume that statistics generated in a particular area are representative of the country as a whole; many other factors may be involved. Researchers must ask what the medical practices are in such areas. Are intensive surveys being carried out? Are cases being more accurately reported to the various tumor registries?

Experts are currently looking into the estrogen-cancer situation. They are finding that a number of other factors which might affect the results are not reflected in the studies reported to date. One such factor is the possibility that the rate of *cancer detection* has been increased for certain medical conditions. For example, since estrogen therapy may be associated with vaginal bleeding, the care of any patient with such bleeding requires careful diagnostic study. The result of the study may show that a cancer is present. At this point it is possible to draw two different conclusions: (1) that estrogen caused the cancer or (2) that the patient already had a precancerous condition or an early cancer and it was the bleeding produced by the estrogen which prompted the diagnostic procedures. What suggests the second conclusion is that the studies also showed that the women who were treated with estrogen had less advanced tumors than those who were not. This "screening" phenomenon has appeared on other occasions. When the first mass surveys for cervical cancer were done using Papanicolaou smears, there was a sharp increase in the number of cervical cancer cases. This was also true when public health programs aimed at detecting diabetes and hypertension were carried out. During the early years of screening for any disease, the incidence will *appear* to go up, but this is due to the increased detection of the disease. We now know that statistically the incidence then begins to decrease and continues to do so as the earlier forms of cancer are cured and, therefore, the later forms do not develop. There is a possibility that we are witnessing the same situation in relation to the increased incidence of cancer of the endometrium.

In addition to the "screening" phenomenon, the nature of the control groups may be a confounding factor. In one study, there were distinct differences between the women studied for endometrial cancer and the women chosen for controls. The majority of the endometrial cancer patients were middle-class, frequently obese, older white women, a group known for years to have a much higher rate of cancer of the endometrium. Many of the women chosen as controls had cervical cancer, a disease that occurs most frequently in younger women of lower socioeconomic groups. Therefore, were these good comparison groups? It is difficult to know. Furthermore, two of the studies excluded from consideration a large group of women who had previously had hysterectomies. It would be useful to know whether their hysterectomies were for cancer and whether or not these women had been taking estrogen. In 1967, a study carried out with a properly controlled group—matched for age, socioeconomic status, number of children and abortions, weight, contraception, menstrual history, diabetes, and high blood pressure—showed no difference between the frequency of endometrial cancer in the women who had received estrogen and those who had not. Although this study does not refute the FDA data, it does point out that all studies do not lead to the same conclusion.

A few years ago, studies appeared suggesting that reserpine (a drug used to treat hypertension) caused breast cancer. The reporting of these studies by the media produced the same sort of general consumer anxiety we are seeing today in relation to estrogen. In the case of reserpine, the verdict was reversed a few years later when better studies were carried out, but much damage had already been done. Estrogen may turn out to be safer than we think or riskier, but the data we have now are not conclusive.

A MUTUAL DECISION

Clearly, for those women who have a definite medical need for estrogen therapy, the risk versus benefit ratio must be weighed carefully. Undoubtedly, new studies will be appearing on the question of whether or not estrogen is safe to use. If you have questions about these new conclusions, you can expect your doctor to tell you whether the latest studies are well designed and well carried out; if the studies are valid, your doctor should interpret how the new information affects the treatment you are about to receive if it includes a therapeutic trial of estrogen. The decision to take estrogen or not to take estrogen is a mutual decision you make *with* your doctor.

> Lucinda B was a fifty-one-year-old upper-middle-class woman who went through her menopause three years ago. She came in complaining of nervousness, a constant sense of foreboding, and a general feeling of unhappiness. She had no specific physical problems and appeared to be in excellent health. She had four children, the first three married and the fourth away at school. Her husband was a very successful hard-working businessman who traveled a great deal. She had a lovely home and several servants, and could buy anything she wanted. She found that she was eating too much and gaining weight, drinking more and starting earlier in the day. She had no real interests or hobbies. She wanted a prescription for estrogen because a number of the women in her bridge club told her it would help solve her problem. Only with considerable difficulty was it finally possible to get her to accept

the fact that estrogen would be of no help to her. Only then was it possible to attack her problems on a basis more difficult for her to accept but ultimately more helpful.

BEFORE YOU TAKE ESTROGEN

There are certain basic evaluations your doctor must make before you receive estrogen therapy. He or she will take a detailed history, perform a careful physical examination, and take blood and urine specimens as well as a Pap smear to send to the laboratory. This, of course, is really no different from the ordinary routine usually carried out prior to the treatment of any other gynecological disorder and simply represents good standard medical practice. Your doctor will want to rule out any conditions (discussed later in this chapter) that would make it inadvisable to take estrogen. Before prescribing estrogen treatment, your doctor must establish that you have a condition for which estrogen is effective. Your doctor should describe to you what to expect from the use of the drug, giving both the positive benefits and the more common side effects such as nausea, and vomiting. Your doctor should caution you about the unusual but potentially dangerous major side effects and the kind of warnings your body will give you: For example, leg or chest pain; headache, particularly if one-sided; or eye symptoms. You must report such symptoms immediately to your physician. Before you begin treatment, you and your doctor will also discuss what kind of follow-up care you are going to have. You can expect to visit your doctor once or twice a year for a breast and pelvic exam, blood pressure, Pap smear, and an assessment of the effectiveness of therapy. Many doctors and clinics have a routine letter and phone call system to remind patients of appointments.

Estrogen, in spite of its current difficulties, is still an effective therapeutic agent, but, like any powerful drug, it must be used carefully under the continued observation of your physician.

WHO SHOULD TAKE ESTROGEN

At one period of time, a few years ago, there was a great vogue for giving estrogen to all women as they approached their menopause and then continuing to give it more or less indefinitely. This school of thought held out the hope that estrogen could keep women looking and feeling young and feminine forever. It has been determined by increased study that this unfortunately is just not the case; estrogen has not proved to be the eternal fountain of youth.

Responsible physicians prescribe estrogen as they do any other powerful drug that carries risks. There must be a very specific medical indication—a problem or symptom for which estrogen is *definitely* effective. The most frequent indication for the use of estrogen is for treatment of the vasomotor symptoms of the menopause, the hot flashes and flushes which may be emotionally and social upsetting to a woman. A second major indication is for the treatment of osteoporosis. Estrogen has been used both for therapy and, by some doctors, for prevention of this bone disease that occurs usually some years after the time of the menopause and can lead to painful and crippling deformities, particularly of the spine. But there is a good deal of debate as to whether estrogen is truly effective in preventing this condition.

Estrogen is also often prescribed for the vaginal changes commonly found when estrogen levels decrease after the menopause. The vaginal tissues become thinner and drier, and some women become unable to have a satisfactory sexual life because intercourse produces pain and irritation. With estrogen treatment, the vagina returns to its more youthful condition. A regular sex life also often helps to keep the vagina youthful.

WHO SHOULD *NOT* TAKE ESTROGEN

There are a number of conditions for which physicians currently rule out, or in medical language *contraindicate*, estrogen therapy. If you have a strong family history of malignancy of the reproductive tract, particularly of the uterus and the breast, you should not take estrogen, since you may increase your risk of getting cancer.

If your physician finds certain problems on pelvic examination, you should not have treatment with estrogen. Benign tumors, fibroids, and polyps may grow under the stimulation of estrogen and produce pain and/or bleeding. If your doctor finds pelvic infection, this would also be a contraindication since you might experience increased bleeding when given estrogen. Women who have undiagnosed abnormal vaginal bleeding should not be treated with estrogen until the cause of the bleeding is diagnosed. Women with endometrial hyperplasia also may tend to develop bleeding more readily when taking estrogen. Since this is a condition which is stimulated by estrogen and which may, in some cases, lead to cancer, estrogen is contraindicated.

If any abnormality of the cervix exists, it must be carefully investigated by Pap smears and biopsies and possibly treated by surgery and/or cauterization. In this case, estrogen should not be administered until cervical abnormality has been diagnosed and the condition has been successfully treated.

Women who have had vascular disorders such as thromboembolism, cerebrovascular accident, myocardial infarction, and thrombophlebitis should not take estrogen, nor should those with impaired liver function, since the liver is the site of estrogen metabolism.

THE DECISION

Proper treatment of menopausal symptoms includes a careful program of considerate care by the physician, sound diet, adequate exercise, and the referral for psychiatric evaluation if a woman has emotional problems.

Estrogen should be taken only in the following situations:

Answer Yes before You Take Estrogen

1. Do you have any of the following problems?
   a. hot flashes
   b. vaginal atrophy
   c. osteoporosis
2. Are you suffering from your symptoms? Are the flashes frequent, is the atrophy causing pain during intercourse?
3. Have you had a thorough gynecological exam as described in this chapter?
4. Has your doctor discussed the risks and benefits of estrogen therapy with you?

HOW MUCH ESTROGEN?

Estrogen, when prescribed, should be given in the lowest dose effective for the particular medical condition and should be continued only as long as the need exists. Most doctors recommend that women who have taken estrogen for more than a year have a trial period *without* estrogen to see if symptoms reappear. If they don't, the estrogen may be discontinued.

There are two general approaches to finding out the amount of estrogen a particular woman needs. One approach is to start with a larger dose and, as quickly as possible, taper it off to the lowest dose which is sufficient to control the symptoms. The second approach—and the one which is definitely preferable at this time—is to start treatment with a lower dose, which is raised only if the symptoms are not relieved. Using this method, women may avoid a number of the minor side effects and may receive a lower total dosage.

Estrogen is best administered in a cyclic fashion. Estrogen alone is given for a certain number of weeks to months and is then followed by a period without medication or by a week or so of a progestin. The cyclic method is preferable because there is some evidence that endometrial malignancies are less likely to occur than with noncyclic administration. This is still a greatly debated issue, awaiting further study.

WHAT ABOUT OTHER HORMONES?

Other hormones such as progesterone and androgen have also been found to be useful to some degree in the treatment of menopausal symptoms. The male hormone, androgen, is not as effective as estrogen in the treatment of hot flashes and, since it has a very different biologic function, it does not produce the desired changes in the vaginal mucosa. Some doctors feel that androgen, in conjunction with estrogen, works well in the treatment of osteoporosis. Androgen is also of particular help in treating women who have contraindications (irregular bleeding, fibroids, etc.) to the use of estrogen alone. Some physicians feel that estrogen and androgen, used together, can be given in dosages below the level which would produce side effects if either drug were given alone. Again, further studies are necessary.

Androgen causes side effects when given in sufficient amounts. It will, of course, produce certain masculinizing changes such as acne, deepening of the voice, and the development of the male type of hair distribution. It also tends to produce an increase in body weight because it causes the retention of fluid. If you are taking androgen, you and your doctor must watch for early signs of masculinizing side effects, particularly acne and excessive oiliness of the skin. If the dosage is reduced at this time, there is usually no danger of developing more disturbing and less easily reversed side effects such as hair growth on the face and body.

Androgen may increase a woman's sex drive, probably because of an increased blood supply to the clitoris. Many women taking androgens for the treatment of breast malignancy have noticed not only an increase in sexual desire but also a sense of general well-being.

WHAT KIND OF ESTROGEN?

Researchers have identified three major naturally occurring estrogen compounds which are produced by the ovaries, adrenals and, in pregnant women, by the placenta. The first and the most active compound is estradiol, which is secreted by both the ovary and the placenta. The second, estrone, is somewhat less potent and the third, estriol, is even weaker. It is currently believed that estrone is produced by the ovarian follicle. It is found in the urine of both pregnant and nonpregnant women, in the placenta, and in the adrenal cortex. Estriol has been identified in the urine of pregnant women and in the placenta. A number of other less potent estrogen compounds have also been identified. In a sense, these estrogen compounds produced by a woman's own body are the truly "natural" hormones; the rest are in some way manufactured.

The various estrogen preparations currently on the market fall into two general categories. The so-called natural estrogens are similar to those produced by the body and are derived from the serum of pregnant mares. The synthetic estrogens are substances created in the laboratory. They are not chemically identical to natural estrogen but have comparable estrogenic effects on the body.

Although there is a continuing dispute about the relative value of natural versus synthetic estrogens, there seem to be no basic differences in effectiveness. Both natural and synthetic hormones will relieve symptoms in menopausal women. By and large the "natural" estrogens are better tolerated than the synthetics; they are less apt to produce nausea, vomiting, and headaches. But, any preparation, either natural or synthetic, if given in sufficiently large doses, will produce symptoms.

HOW DO YOU TAKE IT?

Estrogen can be given in a number of different ways, but most women who take estrogen take it by mouth. Certain types of estrogens are more useful than others for a particular route of administration. For example, a number of the natural estrogens such as estrone and estradiol which are very effective when given by injection are ineffective when given orally.

Estrogens may also be administered externally in the form of topical creams, suppositories, and ointments. These preparations are particularly useful for the treatment of symptoms resulting from drying or shrinking of the labia and vagina. They also have the advantage of using less estrogen to treat the symptom than a daily pill. But, even though applied externally, estrogen cream is readily absorbed into the blood stream and therefore may produce the same kinds of side effects estrogen pills do if used in sufficient quantities.

A number of years ago women undergoing surgical menopause were given subcutaneous implants of pellets of estrogens. This technique is not recommended: When a woman experiences difficulties with the drug, the only way to stop treatment is to remove the pellets surgically.

The cost of any medication is an important consideration. By and large the synthetic estrogens taken by mouth are the least expensive, whereas the natural estrogens administered by injection are the most expensive. Currently, estrogens administered by injection are usually limited to those patients whom the doctor wishes to see quite often for medical reasons and to those patients who are retarded or emotionally disturbed and therefore unable to take oral medication reliably.

FOLLOW-UP

Once a woman begins estrogen therapy, it is essential that she receive follow-up care at frequent intervals. One important test is the Pap smear, which shows premalignant and/or malignant changes

70 | THE MENOPAUSE BOOK

in the cervix. Women who are receiving estrogen therapy should have a smear taken approximately every six months.

When vaginal bleeding develops during estrogen therapy, there are two possible reasons: First, it may be withdrawal bleeding due to the estrogen itself. Second, it may be caused by a uterine growth, either benign or malignant. Since the Pap test does not usually reveal what is happening in the uterus, several other diagnostic techniques may be used to determine the cause. A "jet washer" is a relatively new piece of equipment which allows the physician to introduce a solution into the uterus and obtain cells for examination under the microscope. Other methods are endometrial biopsy, which is done in the doctor's office, or a dilation and curettage, which is usually done in a hospital.

The problem of fluid retention is one your doctor will follow because estrogen decreases the amount of salt and water excreted by the kidneys. Excess fluid retention may produce symptoms such as swelling of the legs and feet. A woman who has a cardiac condition may be pushed into cardiac failure by excessive fluid retention resulting from the inappropriate use of estrogen. This accumulation of fluid may also make preexisting epilepsy, asthma, and migraine more severe and may produce breast swelling and tenderness.

Women with preexisting medical problems, while not necessarily unable to take estrogen, must be informed of the potential risks before starting treatment and then watched carefully. For example, women with chronic cardiac and kidney disease may find that their conditions become more difficult to control. Some women find that depression worsens when they take estrogen. Finally, if uterine fibroids exist, they may swell, degenerate, and produce pain as estrogen stimulates them and they outgrow their blood supply.

THE RESPONSIBLE PHYSICIAN

At the present time there is great consternation among women because of the new reports on the adverse effects of estrogen in the medical literature. The hearings at the FDA, its subsequent reports to doctors on the new findings, and the proposed labeling for estrogen have also been made part of the public awareness. Congressional hearings on these topics have added to the outpouring of information. Even more frightening are the articles and reports in consumer magazines and on TV, and the resultant consumer response has been one of severe anxiety. Physicians as well as their patients are concerned.

A few physicians refuse to consider much of this new information seriously and continue to prescribe estrogen freely. Other doctors have completely stopped their use of estrogens because of fear of litigation. Neither of these is a responsible position. Most physicians, however, are concerned about the studies which have been mentioned and will not use these drugs unless there is a specific indication. They are, however, equally concerned about the removal of estrogen from general use since there are certain women who benefit from and need it.

Therefore, this last group of physicians will continue to use this agent only where it is indicated. They will study their patients carefully before treatment, caution them about possible side effects, and tell them what problems to be aware of and what warning signs to report immediately. They will follow their patients carefully, looking for any sign of difficulty. Furthermore, they will attempt to decrease the dose and stop the administration as soon as it is reasonable to do so, based on the patients' response to therapy and their ability to function normally without the continued prescription of estrogen.

5

HYSTERECTOMY

What is a hysterectomy? Before describing the procedure and the reasons for having it done, it is important to get the terminology straight. Because the word *hysterectomy* is often used with great generality, many women aren't entirely sure what's been done to them, what has been removed from their bodies and what remains.

Briefly, hysterectomy, simple hysterectomy, total hysterectomy, and complete hysterectomy all mean the same thing: removal of the entire uterus including the cervix. The ovaries are not necessarily removed. Partial hysterectomy means that the cervix is left in place and only the body or upper portion of the uterus is removed. Radical hysterectomy refers to the removal of the uterus and cervix plus adjacent lymph nodes.

A hysterectomy can save life or greatly improve health; however, a hysterectomy is a major surgical procedure with potentially serious risks and, therefore, should be done only when it is necessary. Unfortunately, it is one of the greatly abused surgical procedures of our time. It has been needlessly performed on women for whom lesser measures would have been adequate. In fact, some of the conditions that would ultimately lead to hysterectomy actually *regress* with menopause, and women who are able to wait may end up avoiding surgery. Women need to understand when this operation is necessary and when it may be of doubtful value. This chapter is an attempt to provide you with specific factual material on hysterectomy for both cancerous and noncancerous conditions. As you read, you will come to recognize that sometimes the decision to have a hysterectomy is not an absolutely black-and-white one. Whatever reasons doctors have for recommending hysterectomy, it is their clear obligation to discuss with you the full facts of your case, the risks involved, and the effects the surgery will have.

BENIGN CONDITIONS THAT *MAY* REQUIRE HYSTERECTOMY

Many of the problems women encounter during the menopausal years are caused by the response of pelvic tissues to changing levels of hormones. Other problems simply reflect changes that occur as cells age.

Fibroids

One of the most common problems seen in women in the later reproductive years (from age thirty onward) is fibroids (leiomyomata uteri). These are benign tumors that grow from the fibromuscular wall of the uterus and tend to be multiple. The signs and symptoms these growths produce depend on their location. Sometimes they cause absolutely no symptoms and are undetectable except by a microscope. If the fibroid is located on the outer surface of the uterus (subserosal) it may grow to a fairly large size within the pelvic cavity. Such a fibroid might not cause symptoms but would usually be detected by the gynecologist in a routine pelvic exam. Because these fibroids may twist, causing pain and internal bleeding, they are usually removed surgically.

If a fibroid is located within the wall of the uterus, it is called intramural and frequently produces enlargement of the uterus, with increased cramping and bleeding during the menstrual period. If it gets to be big enough, it can exert sufficient pressure on the bladder to cause urinary frequency.

If a fibroid is located on the inner surface of the uterus, it is called a submucosal fibroid. Such a fibroid is treated by the uterus as a foreign object—the muscular wall of the uterus contracts and tries to expel the fibroid through the cervix. This, of course, causes severe cramping similar to labor contractions.

Intramural and submucosal fibroids can interfere with the blood supply to the inner lining of the endometrium and cause bleeding. This bleeding shows up externally as abnormally heavy or prolonged menstrual flow. Over months or years, this excessive blood loss can lead to anemia. Intramural and submucosal fibroids can also interfere with the normal development of pregnancy and can account for some cases of infertility.

Fibroids themselves are almost always benign. Most fibroids, particularly intramural ones, are asymptomatic in the early stages and may only be detected during a routine pelvic examination. When fibroids are small and do not cause symptoms or confusing diagnostic signs, such as bleeding, the best thing to do is to leave them alone. Since the growth of fibroids is stimulated by estrogen, they will stop growing and may actually go away by themselves after menopause. Sometimes a fibroid will calcify after menopause. In this case it will not go away but will stay the same size.

Treatment of fibroids is necessary when symptoms are painful and troublesome or when the symptoms suggest the existence of other more serious diseases such as cancer of the endometrium or of the ovary. If a fibroid is causing pain or bleeding, it must be removed. Sudden increase in the size of a fibroid may be a sign of bleeding into the fibroid or, very rarely, may mean the development of malignancy. Rapid increase in size would be a reason to remove a fibroid. An intramural fibroid may also be removed if a woman wants to become pregnant and the location of the fibroid seems likely to affect her ability to conceive.

DIAGNOSING A FIBROID

The first thing the doctor will do is a complete pelvic examination plus a Pap smear. The next step is a D & C, usually performed in a hospital. If the mass or masses cannot be adequately diagnosed by a D & C, a procedure known as a laparoscopy is frequently performed. With the patient under general anesthesia, a tiny incision is made in the umbilicus. Through this a long, narrow lighted tube, the laparoscope, is inserted to examine various organs. If there is still doubt as to the diagnosis, a full exploratory operation, a laparotomy, may be performed. This requires an incision in the abdomen and is considered a fairly major procedure. Further surgery will depend on the location of the fibroid and the problem the woman has been having.

The operation to remove one or more fibroids is called myomectomy. For pedunculated fibroids (those subserosal fibroids growing on a kind of stalk) the operation is usually simple—the fibroid alone is removed, leaving the uterus intact. Intramural fibroids are removed by making an incision in the uterine wall. The problem with excising any individual fibroid is that there is often more than one. If small fibrods are left untouched, they will, of course, grow in the future and may require further operations. But if a woman wishes to become pregnant, small fibroids not causing problems at the moment may be left behind, with no attempt made to remove every single one. A woman who has had an intramural myomectomy must have all future pregnancies delivered by Caesarian section since the uterine wall has been weakened by the incision and the forces of labor could lead to rupture of the uterus.

Once the uterus is removed, fibroids do not recur. Though a woman is no longer able to become pregnant after a hysterectomy, nor will she menstruate, she will *not* experience the symptoms of estrogen deprivation associated with the menopause. Her ovaries continue to provide her with estrogen.

Fibroids are not associated with the formation of tumors, either benign or malignant, of any other organ and do not ever spread to other organs. They are almost never malignant—less than 1 percent will ever become cancerous. Thus, if the doctor makes a definite diagnosis of fibroids, you can be 99 percent sure that yours is a benign condition. If surgery is not necessary initially, regular follow-up is required to detect the development of complications before they become potentially dangerous. With this follow-up, an attitude of watching and waiting is safe.

Endometriosis

Normally, the endometrium (the specialized tissue that lines the inner surface of the uterus) is confined to the inside of the uterus. Sometimes endometrial tissue is present, not only within the uterus but also outside it, attached to the surface of the uterus, ovaries, tubes, bladder, or rectum. This condition is called endometriosis. When endometrium is found within the fibromuscular wall of the uterus itself, it is called adenomyosis. These are benign conditions but they can cause major problems.

No one knows for sure how the endometrial tissue becomes displaced, although there are a number of theories. The most widely held opinion is that during menstruation, the endometrial tissues not only pass through the cervix into the vagina but also back up the Fallopian tubes into the pelvic cavity, where particles implant on the surface lining of the organs in the pelvis: the uterus, the Fallopian tubes, the ovaries, the bladder, and the rectum.

Another theory maintains that the cells of the surface tissues covering the uterus, Fallopian tubes, ovaries, and other pelvic structures retain the ability they once possessed in the embryonic state to differentiate into many types of genital lining cells and that this may occur even in adult life as the result of certain patterns of hormonal stimulation. Although there is evidence to support both of these theories and several others, no one theory explains completely all of the findings and evidence.

The theories are interesting, but endometriosis itself is often a painful problem. Endometrial tissue, even in an abnormal position, continues to respond normally to the fluctuation of ovarian hormones that regulate the menstrual cycle. Just as normal intrauterine endometrium grows and sheds in a cyclic fashion, so does abnormally placed extrauterine endometrium. The latter produces a monthly pattern: a small amount of internal bleeding that causes inflammation and pain. The end result is scarring with formation of blood-filled cysts (chocolate cysts) involving the tubes and ovaries.

Women with endometriosis find that the pain is usually related to the menstrual cycle and is frequently present for some days before their period is due. When the menstrual flow begins, the pain is relieved. Sometimes a very small amount of endometriosis can give rise to very severe symptoms. On the other hand, large cysts and extensive endometriosis may be entirely asymptomatic.

To diagnose this condition, your gynecologist would first perform a pelvic examination just before your period, because this is when the areas of abnormally placed endometrial tissue are most likely to be felt. If cysts have formed, they may cause a pelvic mass that can be detected on pelvic examination at any time of the cycle. Scarring, of course, can give rise to blockage of the tubes and infertility. Depending on the location of the endometrial tissue, it is possible to see bleeding from the vagina between periods or bleeding from the rectum or bladder.

Although these symptoms may strongly suggest the presence of endometriosis, it is necessary to biopsy the tissue in order to differentiate it from other conditions that might be causing the same symptoms, i.e. pelvic infection, uterine fibroids, tubal pregnancy, ovarian cancer, or other pelvic malignancy. The initial step in making a diagnosis is a thorough pelvic examination and biopsy of any tissue that appears to be abnormal in the cervix or vagina. Usually, none is present, and it is necessary to evaluate pelvic nodularity or masses through laparoscopy. Sometimes it is possible to biopsy tissues through the laparoscopy incision, but it may be necessary to make a larger incision (laparotomy) to do a thorough biopsy or to remove large cysts either for further diagnostic tests or because they are threatening to rupture and bleed.

TREATMENT

Treatment of endometriosis depends on the symptoms. If a woman has endometriosis without any pain or bleeding, the only reason to treat the condition would be to allow her to conceive. Otherwise, nothing needs to be done. At menopause, when the ovaries stop manufacturing hormones, the endometrial tissue is no longer stimulated and the condition will regress spontaneously.

When a woman seeks treatment for endometriosis she has two possible choices. The first is hormonal treatment. Endometriosis can be suppressed either by removing the ovaries and thus removing the hormonal stimulation or by suppression with a combination of both ovarian hormones (estrogen and progesterone) at the same time. Because both ovarian hormones are present during pregnancy, pregnancy is one of the best possible treatments when conception is possible. Pregnancy can be simulated by giving hormones in pills that increase in dosage gradually over a period of time—six months to a year. If the treatment is working, there will be no shedding of the endometrium and therefore no periods. If any bleeding from the vagina occurs, then the same thing is happening inside the pelvic cavity and the treatment is not working as it should. If you are being treated for endometriosis, it is important to notify your doctor of any spotting or bleeding so that the dosage level of hormones can be adjusted.

Once the hormone treatment is stopped, menstrual periods return to normal within a few months. Relief of symptoms of endometriosis may last for many years or for only a short time. Unfortunately, there is no way to predict how long it will be, but if a woman is close to menopause, hormone treatment may be a successful permanent solution.

Surgical treatment may also be as temporary in its effects as hormone treatment or it may be permanent. Temporary surgical treatment involves removing all abnormal endometrial tissue that can be seen. Surgery for endometriosis requires a major operation and general anesthesia. Sometimes the abnormally placed endometrial tissue itself is removed, through either excision or cautery, but sometimes there is so much involvement of the uterus, Fallopian tubes, and ovaries that removal of all of the disease requires removal of these organs. After such extensive surgery, a woman faces a dilemma when it comes to seeking treatment for symptoms of estrogen withdrawal; for estrogen may stimulate regrowth of the endometriosis. Some gynecologists believe that if they wait to give hormones for a period of one to two years, such stimulation will not occur. Sometimes estrogen deprivation symptoms can be relieved by giving a combination of hormones. Birth control pills are often prescribed because they will also suppress the growth of any remaining endometrium.

Endometriosis itself is completely benign. In very rare instances, it is possible for cancer to arise in this endometrial tissue, just as it can arise in the endometrium inside the uterus. A woman with endometriosis is not at higher risk for the development of cancer, but since the disease can produce some of the symptoms of cancer (abnormal bleeding, pain, etc.), it is important for a gynecologist to follow anyone with endometriosis closely.

Endometrial Hyperplasia and Polyps

Failure to ovulate and continuous unopposed estrogen stimulation (no interruption with progesterone) causes overgrowth of the endometrium. If this happens throughout the lining, it is called endometrial hyperplasia. If overgrowth occurs in one spot, it is called a polyp. Polyps can also be caused by local irritants such as a retained piece of placenta after pregnancy of any length, an IUD, and infection. With overgrowth of this kind, the endometrium may shed in an irregular fashion, so that instead of having regular menstrual periods—every twenty-five to thirty-five days—a woman will notice irregular vaginal spotting that occurs in a random fashion. The spotting may be very light and only occasional, or it may be continuous or very heavy at times.

Hyperplasia can sometimes but not always be detected on a Pap smear taken from a washing of the uterine cavity. The only nonsurgical way to make this diagnosis is to do a hysterogram—an X-ray study of the inside of the uterus. This study is not a definitive way to make a diagnosis but does assist in directing your physician toward the most abnormal area within the endometrial cavity. Another way of identifying the most abnormal area is hysteroscopy, a procedure in which a thin lighted tube is inserted into the uterus through the vagina so that the endometrium can be looked at directly. This is moderately uncomfortable, causing some cramping.

However they are identified, abnormal areas must then be evaluated with D & C. At the time of D & C it may be possible to tell by the consistency of the inside of the uterus or by the appearance of the tissue that is removed approximately what the problem is, but the final diagnosis will depend on examination of the tissue under the microscope.

Sometimes the only treatment of this condition that is necessary is simple removal of the polyp or the hyperplastic tissue. And since the D & C consists of a scraping out of the lining, this procedure itself may serve as both diagnosis and treatment. If other treatment is necessary, it will usually be hormonal—either progesterone or one of its derivatives is given. Progesterone causes the lining of the uterus to mature; when medication is stopped, the lining is shed, eliminating all abnormal tissue from the inside of the uterus. The uterus may then grow a new, entirely healthy lining. However, the factor that caused the original problem is still at work (for example, failure of ovulation, uninterrupted estrogen therapy, or an ovarian tumor producing estrogen), the process will repeat itself and the endometrial hyperplasia will recur. Since this condition can cause heavy bleeding and anemia, at this point many doctors would recommend hysterectomy. Also, there are certain situations in which the microscopic appearance of the tissue may be premalignant. (In other words, though no cancer is present now, cancer may develop over a period of months or years if the problem is left untreated.) In this case, the doctor may advise a hysterectomy in order to prevent the development of malignancy.

The prognosis for polyps or hyperplasia depends partly on the age of the woman when the symptoms are diagnosed. In a woman who is premenopausal, such a diagnosis is usually benign but may occasionally be premalignant. If a woman is postmenopausal when the diagnosis is made, it is more likely that the problem will be a premalignant one and therefore require a hysterectomy.

Pelvic Relaxation

Another problem that is extremely common in peri- and postmenopausal women is pelvic relaxation. The pelvic organs are well surrounded and supported by fibrous connective tissue, called fascia, which is attached to the bones of the pelvis and holds the organs in place. In some women this tissue is congenitally weak and stretches; in others, advancing age and childbearing account for the loss of elasticity. Obesity, by increasing the pressure on the bladder and the uterus and their supports in the pelvis, will also cause these supports to weaken. Chronic coughing is another possible cause. With gradual weakening of the connective tissue, the bladder, the uterus, or the rectum may gradually drop down into the vagina and eventually may actually protrude from the vagina. The woman with a dropped bladder (cystocele) may have trouble holding her urine when she coughs or sneezes or lifts heavy objects. Relaxation of the rectum (rectocele) may be aggravated by constipation and may also give rise to additional constipation since, when the woman bears down to move her bowels, the pressure is directed toward the front wall of the rectum rather than toward the anal opening. Though many women have difficulty with urination or bowel movement, it is possible for a woman to be totally asymptomatic except for a feeling that something is protruding from the vagina.

It is usually easy to diagnose these conditions on physical examination. Since there are other possible causes for urinary incontinence, it is also important to have a more detailed evaluation of the urinary tract. Such an evaluation would include a dye study of the kidneys, known as an intravenous pylogram (IVP), and an examination of the inside of the bladder, called cystoscopy. Both are very simple and painless examinations. The IVP consists of injecting a liquid that is opaque to X rays into a vein in the arm. (The injection is the only uncomfortable part of the exam.) After the injection, X rays are taken of the kidneys and bladder as they excrete the dye. Cystoscopy, a painless examination that feels no different from a catheter, is an examination of the inside of the bladder. Occasionally there is the slight discomfort of feeling the need to urinate, but this is never painful.

Once other possible causes of the urinary incontinence have been ruled out, the first treatment for cystocele usually consists of doing exercises to tighten the muscles of the pelvic floor so that they will give support to the bladder and other pelvic structures. These exercises are called "Kegel's exercises." At first, the patient attempts to stop urination in midstream. This may not be possible in severe cases, but even the attempt to stop urination will begin to give tone to weak muscles. With time and concentration it will be possible to accomplish this goal. Once the feeling of contracting these muscles is familiar to a woman, she can then contract them at any time, day or night, when she has a free moment. These contractions should be done five to ten times per session, with relaxation after about three to five seconds. When the muscles become stronger, it is possible to tighten them before coughing and therefore prevent the loss of urine at the time of coughing. These exercises must be kept up indefinitely. If they work, surgery can be avoided.

If Kegel's exercises are not successful in controlling stress incontinence, then a pessary is sometimes recommended. Unfortunately, this is usually not very effective and can cause irritation.

Many surgical procedures have been devised to correct the problem of urinary incontinence, but the multiplicity of procedures reflects the fact that no one operation is perfectly successful. Some involve supporting the bladder by suspending it from the inside of the pubic bone. Others involve tightening the neck of the bladder. In most cases it is impossible to control the incontinence and keep the bladder suspended without removing the uterus. Therefore, a hysterectomy is usually part of the corrective surgery for this problem. If a hysterectomy is not done, the incontinence will certainly recur, sooner or later. Even though a hysterectomy is done, there is still a chance that the problem will recur, and this is particularly true if the underlying cause of the incontinence has not been corrected. In certain cases, such as congenital weakness of the pelvic connective tissue, it may be impossible to correct the underlying problem. If chronic coughing is an underlying cause, then the woman needs to give up smoking or have her pulmonary disease treated. If obesity is at fault, then the answer is obviously weight loss. Because surgery has a poor chance of succeeding if these problems are not brought under control, most doctors will refuse to do any surgery until they have been dealt with. Even under the best of circumstances, surgical cures may not be permanent and another surgical procedure may be necessary within a few years.

CANCEROUS AND PRECANCEROUS CONDITIONS OF THE GENITAL TRACT

The word *cancer* is a frightening one, associated in our minds with wasting and death. And any mention of cancer frequently arouses so much anxiety that we are almost afraid to talk about it.

In 1975 two prominent women with breast cancer, Betty Ford and Happy Rockefeller, talked openly with the press about their disease. In 1976 the treatment of Senator Hubert Humphrey for bladder cancer stimulated a similar frank discussion of the treatment of another type of cancer. The willingness of these individuals to speak up, combined with strong American Cancer Society educational campaigns, has helped enormously to make cancer a subject of public discussion. Women have become more aware of early symptoms and more able to bring them to their doctors' attention.

Even before symptoms occur, precancerous conditions may be discovered and treated early enough to prevent cancer itself from occurring. These premalignant conditions produce no symptoms and can only be detected if a physical examination and Pap smear are done. Even if cancer has begun to develop, catching it at the earliest possible stage allows the majority of women to be cured.

Cancers of the female genital tract account for 14 percent of all cancer for women of all ages and 30 percent of the cancers diagnosed in women thirty-five to fifty-five years of age. Seventy-five percent of these cancers arise in the cervix and endometrium and 25 percent arise in the ovaries.

When Dr. George Papanicolaou first developed his method for examining the cells shed from the cervix and vagina (the Pap smear), it was intended to determine the existence of cancer itself. Some years later, it became evident that the Pap smear detected not only cancer but precancerous conditions as well. We learned that the vast majority of cancers of the cervix were preceded by a continuum of abnormalities that were similar but lesser in degree—varying from dysplasia (mild, moderate, or severe) to *carcinoma in situ* (a term used to refer to cells that look just like cancer cells but that do not yet have the ability to invade adjacent tissues or to spread to other parts of the body). After years of observation, it has become clear that untreated dysplasia will progress to carcinoma in situ, which, if left untreated, will develop into cancer that can spread. If treated completely these problems will neither develop into cancer nor recur in the treated area.

A New Term: CIN

Recently, a single term has come to encompass all degrees of this premalignant disease process—*cervical intraepithelial neoplasia* or CIN. CIN does not cause symptoms and can be detected only by Pap smear. There are certain characteristics shared by women who are likely to develop CIN that can be used to identify high-risk individuals. Although at one time researchers thought that circumcision of the male sexual partner protected against the development of CIN and cervical cancer, this is no longer believed to be true. The only factors that we now consider crucial are early age at first sexual intercourse, early age at first childbirth, multiple childbirths, and multiple sexual partners. It is believed that some substance transmitted through sexual activity comes into contact with the cervix at a time when the lining tissues are particularly susceptible. Many culprits have been named over the years including smegma (the debris that collects under the foreskin of the uncircumcised male), certain bacteria, parasites, and a a virus: herpes simplex type II. All have been studied extensively, without conclusive results. Even though sexual activity is necessary to develop this problem, it is clear that the vast majority of sexually active women do not get it. Obviously, some other factor or group of factors must be involved. It is clear that avoidance of sex is not a solution to the problem. Therefore another means of control must be found.

That control is best provided at the present time by having regular Pap smears, which will detect any kind of cell change. If CIN is present, it can be evaluated by a microscopic examination of the cervix (called colposcopy), which can be performed in the doctor's office. This procedure outlines the extent of the lesion and allows a biopsy to be taken from the most abnormal area. Biopsies usually feel like a quick pinch but may be completely painless. The colposcopic examination itself involves no more discomfort than a Pap smear.

Treatment will depend, first of all, on how severe the condition is. Other factors that will be involved in determining the kind of therapy will be the age of the woman, her desire for childbearing, her general medical condition, and finally, how complete an evaluation was performed through colposcopy.

If evaluation is complete, and the gynecologist has been able to see and evaluate the entire lesion, treatment is the next step.

TREATING CIN

CIN can be effectively treated in the doctor's office. Three major methods are now used as outpatient treatment: cryotherapy (a freezing procedure), electrocautery (burning), and CO_2 laser treatment. In each method, the top layer of abnormal cells is killed and healing proceeds with replacement by normal cells. Only one treatment is necessary in 80 to 90 percent of all cases. In another 10 to 20 percent a second application may be necessary.

Surgical methods of treatment include cervical cone biopsy and hysterectomy. Hysterectomy is the ultimate cure and may be used in more advanced cases such as severe dysplasia or carcinoma in situ if a woman is not interested in having any more children. Hysterectomy for this condition would not require removal of the ovaries.

Cone biopsy is an operation to remove the central portion of the cervix, leaving the uterus intact. It is done through the vagina and therefore requires no major incision. It is performed in a hospital, using general anesthesia. The risks involved (still less than the risks of hysterectomy) make this a procedure best done only if colposcopy has proven unsatisfactory. Heavy bleeding may occur either immediately or at any time up to about two weeks after conization. Removal of such a large portion of the cervix may also affect childbearing ability. The major advantage of conization is that it not only makes complete diagnosis possible but it may also remove all of the disease in the same step. It cannot be considered a minor procedure, but it is certainly less traumatic than a hysterectomy. It is particularly important in the treatment of a woman who desires further childbearing.

The prognosis for CIN is excellent if it is treated properly and if follow-up is adequate. Under these conditions the cure rate for CIN should be 100 percent. If the more conservative methods of treatment such as cryotherapy or electrocautery are used, follow-up care must be regular and prolonged, with visits every four to six months over a one- to two-year period. It is also important to realize that though the area treated may be completely cured, a woman who has had CIN in the cervix still has a 3 to 4 percent chance of developing a similar but separate lesion in the vagina or the vulva at some time in her life. Pap smears are therefore still a necessary part of preventive health care for these women.

If CIN is left untreated, it will eventually become cancer. The amount of time required to progress to cancer depends on the degree of severity of the lesion. Carcinoma in situ is estimated to take from one to five years to develop into invasive cancer. Moderate dysplasia, on the other hand, will take anywhere from five to twenty years to progress to become cancer. An occasional case will progress more rapidly, so treatment should not be deferred any longer than is absolutely necessary to establish an accurate diagnosis. What is so encouraging for women is that the majority of cervical cancers can be prevented by treating CIN. If every woman who has ever been sexually active were to obtain a regular Pap smear, cervical cancer could be almost completely eliminated as a disease. And, in fact, this has happened in one part of the United States. This is Jefferson County, Kentucky, where an intensive Pap smear screening program has been carried out over the past two decades. Prior to the program, there was a high incidence of cervical cancer. Now the disease is practically unheard of except for women who have moved into the county very recently and were therefore never screened before.

Cancer of the Cervix

As we've seen, cancer of the cervix is often an avoidable disease. It is also usually curable. At this time, it is the second most common genital cancer in American women. It accounts for 11 percent of all cancers in women of all ages and for 30 to 40 percent of all malignant tumors of the female reproductive tract. Two percent of all women will develop cancer of the cervix at some point in their lifetime. There are 30,000 new cases diagnosed each year and 13,000 women die yearly of this disease. Cancer of the cervix is most common in women between the ages of twenty-five and fifty-five, but it can be seen from the teen-age years into the late nineties. Less than 5 percent of women with cervical cancer are in their teens while about 15 percent are in their twenties. The incidence curve rises gradually into the late forties and then remains stable and gradually falls off in the eighties and nineties.

As we discussed in the section on CIN, at one time or another just about everything has been related to the development of CIN and cervical cancer. The one statistical finding that has been consistent is that women who develop cervical cancer tend to have had sexual intercourse at an early age as measured by age at first marriage and age at first pregnancy. When a woman begins intercourse at age fifteen to nineteen, her chances of developing cervical cancer are two times greater than if she begins after the age of twenty. Childbearing at less than age fifteen increases the mother's chance of developing cervical cancer threefold. More than four pregnancies or multiple sexual partners also increase the risk.

Socioeconomic status is another factor increasing the risk of developing cervical cancer, with lower-income groups having a much higher risk than middle- and upper-income women. Racial influences are also possible since black women are almost twice as likely to develop cancer of the cervix as are white women. However, this may not be a direct effect of race but rather a reflection of the current economic status of blacks in the United States.

In the past, Jewish women have had a markedly lower incidence of cervical cancer—less than one-fifth that of the rest of the population. At one time it was thought that circumcision helped protect Jewish women from cervical cancer, but this view is not supported by recent detailed epidemiologic studies. The decreased risk was probably related to the fact that, in the past, marriage under the age of twenty, multiple sexual partners, and large numbers of children were uncommon in the Jewish culture.

Women whose mothers took DES (diethylstilbesterol, a synthetic estrogen) during pregnancy to ward off miscarriage, and who were therefore exposed to the chemical *in utero*, are at risk for a very rare form of cervical and vaginal cancer. This drug was widely used in the 1940s and 1950s, so that the oldest members of this particular group are now in their mid-thirties. Fortunately, relatively few cases (a worldwide total of 250 by 1975) have been reported although millions of women took the drug. Any exposed woman should be examined regularly starting about one year after onset of menstrual periods or by age fourteen. More detailed information for exposed women can be obtained from the U.S. Department of Health, Education, and Welfare by requesting booklet number (NIH) 76-1118.

TREATMENTS

Treatment of cancer of the cervix depends on the stage of the disease. The two major alternatives are surgery and radiation therapy. The extent of the surgery depends on the location and extent of the disease. If the malignancy is what is termed "microinvasive," then a simple hysterectomy may be adequate treatment. If the tumor is still small but more deeply invasive, then a radical hysterectomy with removal of the tissues adjacent to the cervix and all of the lymph nodes that drain the cervix would be the treatment of choice. In both operations, the ovaries may or may not be removed depending on the age of the woman.

For most other cases, radiation therapy is the usual treatment. Such radiation is given in two parts. The first consists of external treatments, which are painless and are given on a daily outpatient basis for a period of a month to six weeks. The second portion of the treatment is given as either a radium or a cesium implant in the hospital. Applicators containing the radioactive element are placed inside the uterus, usually under anesthesia. The length of time the implant is left in place will range from one to three days and varies with the dose that is to be given. No anesthesia is required for removal of the applicators. All such implants are carried out within the hospital.

Some tumors that are still localized to the pelvis but that involve the bladder or the rectum may also be treated surgically. In such cases, it may be necessary to remove either the bladder or the rectum or both. If the rectum is removed it is because tumor involves that structure and would soon make normal functioning through it impossible. A colostomy is created and this allows the woman both to be cured of her cancer and to be able to eliminate waste products safely. If the bladder is removed, an artificial bladder is made from an isolated loop of small bowel, and normal kidney function can be maintained while saving the life of the woman. This operation is the one that was used in treating Senator Hubert Humphrey.

The prognosis after treatment of cervical cancer depends of course on the extent of the disease at the time of treatment. Most of the world's major medical centers report survival statistics in five-year terms. This is because long-term follow-up of those women who survive for five years reveals that very few will ever have recurrence of their cancers after that time. The five-year cure rate for Stage I cancer of the cervix is about 85 percent, for Stage II about 65 percent, for Stage III about 35 percent, and for Stage IV about 20 percent.

Follow-up examinations in cancer of the cervix, as in any cancer, are exceedingly important and should be very frequent for the first two years. Generally, women are seen every two to three months in the first year, every three to four months in the second year, and every six months thereafter. Routine follow-up studies such as chest X ray and IVP (kidney X ray) are usually performed at regular intervals. Pap smears are of course done at each visit. The reason for such close follow-up is that this affords the best opportunity to catch and treat any recurrence or any new lesion at the earliest possible time. In addition, any potential complications of the treatment can be prevented or treated early.

Endometrial Cancer

Just as cancer of the cervix has a premalignant stage, so does endometrial cancer (cancer of the lining of the uterus). Although endometrial hyperplasia is *not* a malignant condition, it may progress to one; therefore, it must be evaluated and followed carefully—and often treated.

Cancer of the endometrium is the second most common malignancy of the female genital tract in the United States. It occurs most often in peri- and postmenopausal women, with the greatest number of cases occurring in the late forties, the fifties, and the early sixties. However, younger women do get this disease. About 20 percent of cases occur in women under the age of forty. It is very uncommon under the age of thirty.

Endometrial cancer is more common in women who have never borne children, though whether there is some third factor both preventing pregnancy and allowing development of the cancer is not clear. It is generally believed that an excesss of estrogen stimulation unopposed by progesterone has something to do with the development of endometrial cancer. Women who have anovulatory cycles (thus lacking progesterone reversal of the estrogen that stimulates growth of the endometrium) have an increased risk of developing cancer in the endometrium. In addition, before such cancer develops, a pattern of endometrial hyperplasia will often be observed. Another bit of evidence that points toward estrogen as one of the contributing factors is the increased incidence of this disease in women who have ovarian tumors that secrete estrogen. Finally, there is recent evidence indicating that women who develop endometrial cancer are more likely to have taken estrogen at some time in their lives than women who do not get the disease.

Still, estrogen is only one factor. Clearly, not all women who have unopposed estrogen or who take estrogen will develop endometrial cancer. There are many other factors that must be involved and are as yet unidentified; some may relate to genetic predisposition, others may have something to do with the balance of various kinds of estrogens in the woman's body.

The first sign of endometrial cancer is almost always abnormal vaginal bleeding; that is, bleeding between periods, increased length of the period, or bleeding after menopause. Diagnosis is accomplished first by a pelvic exam and a Pap smear. An ordinary Pap smear will reveal the presence of endometrial cancer only occasionally. The reason for the low yield rate is that the Pap smear is taken from the vagina and the outside of the cervix where the tissues can be wiped for cell samples. It is somewhat more difficult to take a sample of the cells wiped from the *inside* of the uterus. This can be done by using a special technique in which a thin tube is inserted into the endometrial cavity and cells are either wiped or washed off the lining. This kind of procedure increases the positive rate to 70 or 80 percent when properly performed and evaluated. However, since it is a mildly uncomfortable procedure for most women it is not a useful tool for screening. The diagnosis of endometrial cancer must be made on the basis of tissue samples taken from the inside of the uterus at D & C (dilatation and curettage). This procedure is done with anesthesia, either local or general, and is considered a minor operation.

Staging of endometrail carcinoma is an important step in determining treatment and prognosis. Stage I endometrial cancer is confined to the uterine body; Stage II involves the cervix; Stage III involves other pelvic structures; and Stage IV involves the bladder, the rectum, or structures outside of the pelvis such as the lung or bone. About 70 percent of all endometrial cancers are in Stage I when first diagnosed.

Treatment is usually a combination of radiation and surgery for earlier stages. Unless a woman is medically unable to tolerate surgery, a hysterectomy will almost always be performed in Stages I and II—with radiation therapy frequently added before surgery to reduce the size of the tumor and to kill cancer cells that may have spread beyond the uterus. When widespread disease is present, progesterone may also be added to the treatment regimen. Fortunately progesterone is a form of chemotherapy that has very few side effects and is almost universally well tolerated. In addition, it has an effectiveness rate of about 30 percent—that is, in about one out of three cases the disease will be controlled or eliminated. Usually progesterone must be continued for the rest of a woman's life, since stopping may allow regrowth of suppressed cancer cells.

Cure rates for endometrial cancer are reasonably good. In Stage I, which accounts for about two-thirds of all cases, the cure rate is about 75 percent. In Stage II it is about 50 percent; in Stage III it is about 30 percent; and in Stage IV it is about 15 percent. Although these results are favorable when compared with other cancers such as those arising in the lung or the stomach, a major effort is now being directed at improving the cure rate through earlier diagnosis and better treatment.

Ovarian Cancer

Ovarian cancer is the third most common malignancy of the female genital tract in the United States, with 17,000 new cases diagnosed each year. It accounts for 25 percent of genital malignancies and 9 percent of all malignancies in American women of all ages. Eleven thousand deaths occur annually, making ovarian cancer the fourth most common cause of cancer death in women, exceeded only by cancers of the breast, colon, and lung.

RISK

As is true in any malignancy, early diagnosis is the key to a good prognosis. The population at risk for ovarian cancer is generally an older one, since 80 percent of the cases occur after the age of forty and 60 percent of the cases occur after the age of fifty. In fact, carcinoma of the ovary is the most common genital malignancy in women over fifty years of age. Women who have never been pregnant have a somewhat higher risk of developing ovarian cancer. Race seems to be a factor in that the risk in black women is slightly lower than in white or Oriental women. Family history can be important, since family clusters have been seen. In such a situation there may be two or three generations that develop ovarian cancer. Rarely, sisters will develop the disease. Though this is not terribly common, in a family in which such clustering has occurred, all female members should be carefully watched for signs of the disease.

The initial symptoms of ovarian cancer are usually vague: gastrointestinal complaints or abdominal distention related to fluid formation, tumor bulk, or intestinal obstruction. Too frequently, physicians and patients alike may dismiss such vague complaints as "only symptoms of the menopause" and thus delay the diagnosis of ovarian carcinoma. This is easily corrected by making the pelvic examination a part of the initial and routine evaluation of every woman.

What we lack in the battle against ovarian carcinoma is a reliable diagnostic mass-screening test. For the cervix, cytology and colposcopy allow us to detect even premalignant lesions. In the endometrium a D & C will easily lead to diagnosis of malignancy. However, Pap smears taken from the vagina and cervix are rarely positive for cancer of the ovary even when advanced disease is present. Fluid aspirated from the pelvic cavity through a needle, can be examined for tumor cells, but this procedure is not practical for screening large numbers of women. Pelvic examination remains the only good indicator of problems, even though it is still difficult to feel very early tumors.

In the past few years, an international staging system has been developed. This system is based on the tumor spread as revealed by surgical and microscopic findings. In Stage I the tumor is limited to the ovaries; in Stage II uterus and tubes or surfaces of other pelvic structures such as the rectum or the bladder are involved; Stage III indicates involvement of other abdominal structures such as the surfaces of the small bowel or liver; and Stage IV indicates tumor spread outside the abdominal cavity or deep within the liver, bladder, or rectum.

Since the internal location of the ovaries makes early diagnosis difficult, a very high percentage of cases are quite advanced at the time of initial identification. Most centers report that 50 to 60 percent of their cases are in Stage III when they are initially seen. The problem is of course to shift the number of cases in Stage III to lower stages by earlier diagnosis. The inability to do this accounts partially for the poor record in the treatment of this disease.

TREATMENT

The treatment of ovarian cancer begins with surgical exploration of the abdominal and pelvic contents. The uterus, Fallopian tubes, and ovaries must be removed since these are the most likely organs to be involved with tumor. Next, the omentum, an apron of fat that hangs over the bowels, must be removed since this, too, is frequently involved. Any other tumor bulk that is present is also removed when possible. If any fluid is present in the abdomen, it must be examined for cancer cells. These procedures not only start treatment but also allow accurate staging of the tumor. The single most important prognostic factor in ovarian cancer is the volume of tumor left after surgery. This may reflect the fact that radiation and chemotherapy are more effective with very small volumes of tumor. About a month after surgery, any additional treatment that is prescribed will be given. This may include radiation therapy and/or chemotherapy, with the amount depending on the extent of the disease.

Survival statistics in ovarian cancer are dismal, with an overall five-year survival rate of only 25 percent. This is largely because most patients have advanced disease when first diagnosed. In addition to inaccessibility of the ovaries for examination, one of the major reasons for this poor prognosis is the mode of spread of these cancers. The most common site of early extension is over the surfaces of pelvic and abdominal structures. The surface area available for tumor implantation within the abdominal and pelvic cavity is enormous since it includes the outer covering of the entire bowel. Progression of the disease will lead to multiple areas of intestinal obstruction. Surgical bypass of the obstructed area is possible but the length of bowel available for nutrition is then decreased accordingly. Not only are there potential complications of tumor, but treatment by any method is difficult, since the amount of treatment that can be given is limited by the degree of tolerance of all the intra-abdominal organs, including bowel, liver, and kidneys.

PREPARATION FOR HYSTERECTOMY

Before any surgery is performed, there will be a series of tests that will be required, to make certain both that the treatment is appropriate and that the woman will be able to tolerate the proposed surgery. These will almost always include blood and urine studies and a chest X ray. Frequently an electrocardiogram will be indicated. Other studies that may be involved include ultrasound examination, X rays of the kidneys (intravenous pyelogram or IVP), X rays of the bowels (barium enema), and direct examination of the bladder (cystoscopy) and the rectum (proctoscopy). Other more specialized tests may be obtained before cancer surgery; these include bone scan, hysterogram, lymphangiogram, and upper GI series.

If a woman smokes it is vital that smoking be either eliminated or severely limited for several weeks before major surgery whenever possible. Smokers have a significantly greater rate of postoperative complications such as pneumonia and wound breakdown than do nonsmokers. Obesity is another factor that increases complications and should be brought under control when there is time.

Education is another important part of preparation for surgery that is too often neglected. Misconceptions and myths concerning the proposed surgery should be corrected preoperatively if possible. Review of a pelvic model and thorough discussion of what is and is not being removed will go a long way toward this end. Self-analysis concerning the personal meaning of the uterus, childbearing potential, and menstruation can help outline the changes in body image and self-concept that if left unresolved could lead to an identity crisis. Myths concerning decreased femininity, masculinization, excessive weight gain, accelerated aging, loss of sexual attractiveness, and insanity as a result of hysterectomy must be dispelled.

In all these discussions it is important to include that oft-forgotten third party, the woman's sexual partner. Children also are frequently excluded from preoperative preparation. While details must be varied according to the age and needs of the individual, appropriate explanations should be given to all members of the patient's family whenever possible. Some of this can be done by the physician, but much must be done by the woman herself.

The day before surgery, in the hospital, the patient will be seen by the anesthesiologist, who will discuss with her her past experiences (if any) with surgery and will make a decision about what kind of anesthesia to use. The exact routine of premedication and sedation will be outlined, and any questions about anesthesia will be answered at that time.

HOW IS A HYSTERECTOMY PERFORMED?

A hysterectomy can be done through an abdominal incision or through a vaginal incision. In order to do the hysterectomy vaginally there must be adequate room for the operation. A woman who has never delivered a baby would probably not be able to have a vaginal hysterectomy, whereas a woman who has had several children would be more likely to be able to have her surgery vaginally. If the uterus is enlarged, a vaginal hysterectomy would usually not be possible.

The words that have been used to describe various operations to remove the pelvic organs are sometimes confusing. As was indicated at the beginning of this chapter, the word *hysterectomy* means removal of the uterus—all of the uterus including the cervix. It does not indicate whether or not the tubes and ovaries have been removed.

Unfortunately, many people use the term *partial hysterectomy* to mean that one or both ovaries have been left. Technically, partial or subtotal hysterectomy refers only to the removal of part of the uterus, an incomplete operation that used to be performed when surgical and anesthetic techniques were not as refined and blood-transfusing ability was less competent than it is today. In a subtotal hysterectomy the cervix was not removed and could therefore lead to a recurrence of the problem for which the surgery was done.

None of the operations mentioned so far involves the ovaries. After removal of the uterus, a woman is not able to have children, nor does she have periods. But there is no menopausal syndrome, since the ovaries are still present and ordinarily function normally until the usual age for menopause. As long as one ovary remains, estrogen production will continue, and no menopausal symptoms will appear. Usually, the ovaries are not removed in young women who have many years remaining before natural menopause would occur. The risks involved in many years of estrogen replacement far outweigh the risks of possible development of ovarian cancer or other less dangerous ovarian diseases that might require additional surgery. When a woman reaches her early forties, the years remaining until natural menopause are fewer and the risks become reversed. From this age on, many gynecologists feel that ovaries are best removed at the time of hysterectomy, because a few years of estrogen replacement involve far less risk of major problems than the risks of additional surgery or of possible ovarian cancer. If the ovaries are removed, the procedure is called an oophorectomy. If both ovaries are removed, it is a bilateral oophorectomy, and if the Fallopian tubes (salpinges) are removed along with the ovaries, as is usually done for technical reasons, the procedure is called a bilateral salpingo-oophorectomy. Only if both ovaries are removed will a woman begin to experience the symptoms of estrogen deficiency (so-called surgical menopause), unless of course she has already gone through natural menopause. These symptoms usually first appear within a week after removal of the ovaries and will be alleviated by estrogen replacement therapy if it can be given. Estrogen is never given to women who have had endometrial or breast cancer or who have a strong family history of breast cancer.

A radical hysterectomy involves removal of the tissues between the cervix and the pelvic wall. This is much more difficult, since the ureters (the tubes that carry urine from the kidneys to the bladder), the bladder, and the rectum must be carefully dissected free from these tissues. This is an operation that is done for cancer and is almost always performed by a specialist trained in gynecologic cancer surgery. Removal of the lymph nodes in the pelvis (lymphadenectomy) usually accompanies a radical hysterectomy and is also performed by the cancer specialist.

Additional cancer surgery, which may be performed in certain rare instances when cancer has spread only to the bladder or the rectum, includes removal of those diseased organs with additional procedures for diverting the urinary stream or the fecal stream to separate openings in the abdominal wall. These are extreme measures and are usually performed by gynecological cancer specialists, but they may also be performed by general surgeons or genitourinary surgeons who are specially trained in cancer surgery.

AFTER A HYSTERECTOMY

Whatever type of hysterectomy is done, there will be pain from the incision. This lasts a day or two and is treated with pain medication to keep it under control. Doctors and nurses should encourage the patient to cough to keep her lungs cleared out and to exercise her legs so that phlebitis does not develop. Most doctors prefer to get their patients out of bed as soon as possible after surgery so that peneumonia and phlebitis can be avoided. Because bowels temporarily do not move fluid along after the abdominal cavity has been entered, it is not possible to eat for several days after such surgery; therefore, intravenous fluids are given. Gradually the bowels regain their function, and as they start to do this—on the third or fourth day—there will be abdominal cramping. This cramping usually lasts no longer than twelve to twenty-four hours. Most patients are sufficiently recovered from the immediate effects of the operation and are eating and moving around well enough at the end of one week to go home and continue their recuperation there. The return of strength is usually slow but steady; most women feel able to resume a full load of normal activity after about four to six weeks. However, it may take up to six months to feel normally energetic, and the older a woman is at the time of surgery, the longer this period of extended recovery will take.

Healing itself takes many months to be complete. The incision is strong enough to allow removal of the skin sutures after about one week. It is possible to observe the external signs of healing by looking at the scar. Initially after an operation, the scar will be red. As more scar tissue is laid down, the appearance of the scar gradually changes to white. This process takes many months, and as it progresses the scar becomes even stronger.

During recovery from surgery, the diet should contain plenty of proteins, fresh fruits, and vegetables. Because of decreased activity levels it is easy to gain weight if overall intake of carbohydrates and fats is not limited. As activity increases back to preoperative levels, so can the diet. As always, weight gain is the result of imbalance in the ratio of intake and output. With a little care in diet planning, weight gain need not follow surgery.

Similarly, flabby muscles secondary to the inactivity following surgery can be gradually retoned by exercises. It is usually safe to begin conditioning exercises by four to six weeks postoperatively. They should be started very slowly and increased only gradually, always remembering that muscles that have been inactive for some time are more subject to strain.

Psychological changes after hysterectomy will depend to some extent on a woman's self-image and what it means to her to be able to bear children. There are some changes, however, that are common to all people who undergo any major stress including surgery. In the first day or two, the person is usually preoccupied with simple matters of keeping comfortable and of being glad that everything is over. On about the third to the fifth day there will be a letdown reaction, sometimes known as the "third-day blues." Weeping for no obvious reason and feelings of sadness are normal and should be expressed.

This "blue period" may be aggravated by certain factors in an individual's personality that give the surgery special meaning to her. It is wise to try to identify these factors prior to surgery so that they may be understood and dealt with.

Sexual functioning will obviously be temporarily curtailed due to the physical limitations of recent surgery. However, alternate methods of sexual gratification can be substituted for intravaginal intercourse once the immediate postoperative period is past and interest in sex returns. By the time six to eight weeks have passed, intravaginal sexual activity is usually possible, but it may be many months before completely normal sexual functioning returns. It is important to remember that physical factors are not the only (nor even the major) determinants of sexual gratification. The trauma of a life-threatening situation, the loss of emotionally significant organs, changes in body image, and the attitudes of sexual partners will all have profound effects on sexual functioning. These effects are normal, and when dealt with openly, they will be transient. If allowed to go unexpressed and unexplained, they will fester and become a chronic source of problems.

UNNECESSARY SURGERY

Volumes have been written about unscrupulous or careless physicians who take advantage of their patients by recommending surgery that is not really indicated. The best way for you to avoid this kind of problem is to be aware of some of the reasons for surgery and their importance and to ask plenty of questions about the specific reasons for the surgery that is recommended. If you feel that your questions are not adequately answered, it is a good idea and well within your rights to obtain a second opinion from a physician you trust. A trusted family physician or your local County Medical Society will be able to provide you with names of qualified ethical physicians who can provide you with a second opinion.

Another way of decreasing the possibility of unnecessary surgery is to choose the doctor least likely to give you bad advice. Physicians who are board-certified in obstetrics and gynecology have passed both written and oral examinations that require of them established levels of knowledge and standards of practice. One of the things that the American Board of Obstetrics and Gynecology seeks to do is to control unnecessary surgery. If you do not know whether a physician is board-certified, the local County Medical Society will be able to provide you with this information.

In making a decision about whether or not to have an operation of any kind, the major caution that you should observe is to avoid delaying *necessary* surgery for too long. You should also remember that there is usually more than one way to treat most problems, and that the solution for you may be very different from that for someone else. All aspects of your situation—social, economic, and psychological, as well as medical—must be considered. A thorough exploration of all these factors will allow you and your doctor to come to a decision together. This process can produce a mutual respect and trust that can only lead to better and more complete medical care.

6

BREAST CANCER

Why a chapter on breast cancer? Unlike most of the other chapters in this book, this one does not have a direct bearing on the subject of menopause. Nevertheless, it is an important concern to women at this time of life, for the risk of breast cancer increases after the age of forty. Unfortunately, some women, in an effort to deny the possibility, do not have regular breast exams or perform self-examinations. Here we intend to give as much reassurance as possible to the woman who discovers or fears discovery of a lump in her breast. Breast cancer is a treatable, curable disease, especially in its early stage, before it has spread beyond the breast. Even without early detection, one point that must be emphasized is that a woman with more advanced cancer may be helped greatly.

WHO IS AT RISK?

Breast cancer occurs rarely in women under twenty, but between the ages of thirty and fifty there is a rapid rise in the risk of developing the disease. Although the incidence tapers off at around sixty, it continues to increase until a woman is eighty years old. At this age the woman's probability of developing breast cancer is twice as high as when she was sixty.

Some women have a significantly lower risk of developing breast cancer. For example, those who have undergone a hysterectomy and a bilateral oophorectomy (removal of both ovaries) before age forty have one-fourth the risk of developing breast cancer. The risk is lower for women who have multiple pregnancies or whose first pregnancy occurs before the woman is twenty years old. Incidence of breast cancer varies in different countries and is particularly low in Japanese and Middle-Eastern women. There is also a low incidence in non-Caucasians and in women of a low socio-economic status. Some researchers have hypothesized that this may be due to the diet; there seems to be a connection between a higher intake of animal fats and a higher incidence of breast cancer. In countries where dietary animal fat is very low, there is a very low incidence of breast cancer.

Some of the factors that increase the risk of breast cancer are related to genetics, exposure to radiation, and certain aspects of childbearing (women who bear their first child *after* thirty have a somewhat higher risk than average; those who bear their first child in their early twenties have a somewhat lower risk). There is a threefold increase in the incidence of breast cancer among women whose mothers have had breast cancer, and when it does occur in the offspring, it can occur ten years earlier. For example, if the mother had breast cancer at fifty, the daughter could develop the disease at forty. In women who have a genetic predisposition to breast cancer, it occurs in both breasts more often. Exposure to radiation increases the incidence of breast cancer. This fact was sadly demonstrated by the survivors of the atomic bomb dropped on Hiroshima, where the women showed a two- to fourfold increase in breast cancer fifteen years after the explosion. The same delay in occurrence, and also the same increased incidence, is noted in women who have been exposed to excessive X-ray examinations (for TB treatment or evaluation) and in women who were exposed to X-ray treatment to the chest wall for other diseases.

ESTROGENS AND BREAST CANCER INCIDENCE

At the present time, there is no association between birth control pills and an increased risk of breast cancer. It is known that hormonal environment does have an influence on the development of breast cancer. The total amount of estrogen is obviously much higher in women than in men, and the *incidence* of breast cancer is much higher in women than in men. Also, a woman who has had her estrogen supply removed by an oophorectomy has a lower incidence of breast cancer.

There are three major estrogen compounds excreted in the urine. One of these compounds, estriol, is decreased in patients with breast cancer. Estriol is increased, however, in patients during the time of pregnancy, especially in women whose pregnancies occur at an early age (early twenties); therefore, some researchers believe that it is estriol that protects women who have had early pregnancies from breast cancer. It is interesting to note that Oriental women have a high estriol level in their urine and, as was previously mentioned, have a low incidence of breast cancer.

DETECTION

Because breast cancer is a treatable, curable disease, especially in its earliest stages, it is obviously important to stress detection. A woman should expect to get yearly breast examinations from the doctor she sees regularly. For most women this will be her gynecologist, but internists and general practitioners are qualified to do the exam—and should include a breast exam as part of their physical evaluation.[1]

SELF-EXAMINATION

The best person to do a breast examination, however, is the woman herself. Women doing self-examinations month after month usually detect a lump or a thickening before a physician could. Those women who are terrified lest they find something can be encouraged by the fact that only 20 to 25 percent of these lumps are going to be malignant. *Seventy-five to 80 percent will be benign!* Approximately 90 percent of breast cancer cases treated by the physician have been discovered by the woman herself.

Breast self-examination should be done once a month. Women who are still menstruating, should do the exam right after they have finished menstruation because that's when the breast is quiescent; estrogen, which before a period makes a woman's breasts tender and lumpy, is at its lowest level after menstruation. Women who have had their

---

1. If your regular doctor does not do breast exams, find one who does.—*Ed.*

menopause should pick an arbitrary date on the calendar and do a self-examination every month on that date. Women who are premenopausal and who have had hysterectomies but not oophorectomies still have ovarian function and produce estrogen; they should try to determine what moods correspond to a postmenstruation frame of mind and set this as the time of breast self-examination.

How to Do a Breast Self-Examination

Start your exam by sitting comfortably in front of a mirror with your breasts completely exposed. What you are looking for is any asymmetry in the breast size that seems different to you from your normal state. Be aware that in many women one breast is normally larger than the other. Look for deviation or asymmetry of the nipples, retraction of the nipple (the nipple looks pulled in), retraction of the skin anywhere along the breast, swelling of the skin, any dimpling of the skin (it may look like the skin of an orange), or any sore. Then raise your arms above your head; look again at the breast for any changes in symmetry. Place your hands on your hips and squeeze your hips so that you are flexing your pectoral muscles. Notice any irregularity in breast contour. After all this, you then lie down. The woman with normal-sized breasts just lies down flat, but a woman with very large breasts lies down with a pillow beneath her shoulder blade on the side she is examining so that her breast is somewhat extended. If, for example, you start with your left breast, use two fingers of your right hand and beginning at the 12:00 o'clock position and starting from the center and moving out, examine the breast in concentric circles. The important thing is to do it very slowly and cover every part of the breast. Younger women have normally lumpier breasts. The first exam should be done with a physician so that he or she may show you what is normal or abnormal.

MAMMOGRAPHY

Mammograms are X-ray studies of the breasts based on the natural contrast provided by the fat content of breasts. As women get older there is more fatty replacement of the breast tissue and therefore mammograms become more accurate in women after age forty. If fine sandlike calcifications appear in the mammogram, then a biopsy is mandatory. These calcifications can be signs of malignancy but the tissue must be studied under a microscope to make a definite diagnosis.

Not everyone, however, should have mammography. The American Cancer Society has established good guidelines as to who should be screened and who should not. A woman at any age who is concerned or whose physician recommends the exam should have one. If a woman is over fifty, annual screening and examinations are advised because the benefits far outweigh the risks. If she is between thirty-five and fifty, she should have one if she has the following risk factors: (1) She has had a previous mastectomy; (2) her mother or sister or both have had premenopausal breast cancer; (3) her mother had postmenopausal breast cancer; (4) she has not borne children; (5) she bore her first child after the age of thirty; (6) she began menstruating at eleven years or under; (7) she has a history of previous benign breast tumors; (8) she has lumps, discharge, or severe pain caused by fibrocystic disease. Women under thirty-five or between thirty-five and fifty with no symptoms and no increased risk should generally not have mammography. For a woman with extremely large breasts, mammography is particularly important regardless of age because it is more difficult to find a lump on physical examination. Women who have previously had cancer in one breast should have yearly mammography on the remaining breast.

The average woman has a 7 percent risk of developing breast cancer in her lifetime. By annually exposing herself to extra radiation, a woman with no particular risk of breast cancer would over a period of fifteen years and after fifteen mammograms increase her risk from 7 to 8 percent.

OTHER TYPES OF SCREENING

A new and superior form of X-ray screening of the breasts is called xerography (or xeroradiography). It uses less radiation to produce a more detailed, reliable, and accurate picture of what is going on in the breast. Unfortunately, the equipment is delicate and often breaks down. Thus, it is still not suitable for mass screening programs.

Thermography, a technique for diagnosing breast changes through differential heat patterns, does not expose the patient to any form of

X-ray radiation. Its great flaw, however, is its inaccuracy. It is positive only 60 percent of the time, leaving 40 percent of cancer cases undiagnosed, and is also falsely positive in 40 percent of normal women.

If You Discover a Lump

The first thing is to have your surgeon examine you. He or she may do a "needle aspiration" under local anesthesia if the lump seems to be a cyst. If a solid mass remains after this procedure, then a more extensive biopsy is necessary.

The most accurate diagnosis of breast cancer depends on microscopic examination, and to have this evaluation done, a surgeon needs to examine tissue from the area where cancer is suspected.

BREAST BIOPSY

Surgical biopsy (rather than outpatient needle biopsy) is preferred for (1) any discrete palpable breast mass, (2) crusted or inflamed lesions of the nipple and bloody nipple discharge, (3) suspicious areas revealed by mammography, and (4) cystic breast masses that have not disappeared or have recurred within one to two months after a cyst aspiration.

Breast biopsy requires admission to the hospital and is best performed under general anesthesia. This is so because lesions are usually deeper within the breast than they appear when being examined by hand manipulation. In addition, the contour of the breast can be more skillfuly restored (if the condition proves benign) and bleeding is better controlled when a patient is under general anesthesia. Breast biopsy is performed through an incision around the dark part of the nipple area (areola). Occasionally, incisions along the natural horizontal lines under the nipple are used. Small drainage tubes are left in place for twenty-four hours after the surgery to prevent collections of blood. In patients with certain other medical problems a needle biopsy under local anesthesia may have advantages.

In the vast majority of cases, the pathologist (the doctor who examines the tissue samples) can make an unqualified diagnosis of benign (75 to 80 percent will be) or malignant from the breast tissue submitted by the surgeon at the time of operation. Occasionally, the situation is more complicated. Under these circumstances a more detailed examination must be made and definitive surgery must be delayed. If mastectomy is delayed for two to four days, it still has as good a chance of being successful as if it were done on the spot.

Many surgeons routinely perform screening tests prior to surgery because a certain percentage of breast cancers may have already spread to distant sites in the body. These tests are designed to reveal sites of spread. Since breast cancer may spread to the lung, liver, and bones, patients receive, preoperatively, a chest X ray, blood tests of liver function (and possibly a liver scan), and X rays (or scan) of the bones. If the diagnosis of cancer is considered very likely, these tests are done before surgery because the presence of disease elsewhere may influence the surgeon's choice of operation.

> For example, a woman has a four-centimeter hard, fixed mass in her breast. The chest X ray shows evidence of tumor spread to the lungs. The surgeon will probably not do a radical mastectomy because this procedure is designed to remove tumor that has spread only as far as the axillary nodes (lymph nodes in the armpits). This tumor has clearly spread beyond.

If these tests were not performed preoperatively, then most surgeons would perform them postoperatively as a standard with which to compare future postoperative check-ups. Furthermore, if unsuspected distant spread is found, the physician should be aware of it and suggest suitable treatment: endocrine manipulation, surgery, radiation, or chemotherapy.

STAGING

In order to determine what type of surgery to perform and what kind of postoperative care is desirable, the breast surgeon wants to know how far the disease has spread—whether there is involvement of any of the lymph glands under the arm on the side of the affected breast or whether it has already spread to distant parts of the body. Assigning a "stage" to the cancer is a measure of how far it has spread.

It is generally accepted that breast cancer starts in the breast itself and spreads to the lymph glands which normally drain the breast. These glands are located in the armpit (axilla), under the breastbone (sternum), and under the collarbone (clavicle). The direction in which the cancer spreads is related to its position. If the cancer is in the upper, outer part of the breast, it will spread to the glands in the armpit. If it is in the inner part of the breast it may spread along the internal mammary artery (under the sternum). Studies have shown that two factors increase the possibility of cure: (1) The smaller the original tumor, the greater chance of long-term survival; (2) Tumors that have not spread at the time of detection by the patient or physician are more easily removed, and the patient will usually have a longer survival. Unfortunately, no matter how small or localized the tumor is, small amounts of cancer cells may have already spread by the blood stream to other parts of the body.

What do physicians mean when they talk about Stage I, Stage II, Stage III, and Stage IV? Stage I means that the tumor is less than five centimeters (in some hospitals less than two), that it is not fixed to the chest wall, and that there are no abnormal lymph nodes. Stage II means that the lymph glands are abnormal but movable and the tumor is not attached to the chest wall. Stage III means that either the tumor or the lymph glands are not movable. Stage IV refers to distant spread of the tumor to other areas of the body besides the breast region.

Forty-five percent of breast cancer patients have Stage I cancer when they come to their doctors with a lump; 15 percent have Stage II; 25 percent have Stage III; and 15 percent have Stage IV. The sooner changes or lumps in the breast are detected, the greater the likelihood of its being a Stage I breast cancer.

If women really were examining themselves and picking things up sooner, more of them might be in Stage I. Survival rates vary from place to place. The five-year survival for Stage I is generally 82 percent —82 percent of patients with breast cancer would be alive five years after mastectomy. This is why doctors place a lot of emphasis on self-examination and early detection. Stage II also has a good prognosis. At Memorial-Sloan Kettering (a major cancer research and treatment center in New York City), the five-year survival is also 82 percent for stage II. Stage III survival rates vary from about 48 percent in some places to 61 percent in others. Stage IV has a five-year survival rate ranging from 0 to 12 percent.

WHAT TYPE OF SURGERY IS BEST?

The purpose of any surgical procedure for breast cancer is to remove the entire tumor and cure the patient. Right now, the controversy centers around which procedure will do this for the greatest number of women.

The first successful operation for breast cancer was devised more than a century ago by Dr. Charles Moore in England and it became popularized by a surgeon named Halstead, who did fifty operations and decided this was the appropriate treatment for breast cancer. Halstead gave his name to the procedure still advocated by many surgeons—the Halstead Radical Mastectomy. In recent years, however, this operation has come under increasing criticism by a minority of surgeons and by the public media.

The Halstead radical mastectomy is removal of the entire breast, chest wall muscles (pectoralis major and minor muscles), and all the axillary lymph nodes. The extended radical procedure includes removal of the internal mammary nodes. (The only difference between the two operations is the removal of an extra set of nodes.) Modified radical mastectomy spares the pectoral muscles as well as the interpectoral lymph nodes and, by leaving these muscles intact, offers the patient normal shoulder and arm strength and means that the end result is cosmetically better. The chest wall is not as hollow-looking with the modified procedure.

Simple mastectomy is removal of the breast itself and a few axillary nodes. A partial mastectomy is removal of the skin overlying the tumor and a wide segment of the breast tissue around the tumor. A lumpectomy refers to the removal of the tumor alone.

Numerous studies have tried to compare the long-term survival of women treated with each of the above procedures. Unfortunately there are many defects in the studies, making the interpretation very difficult. Different circumstances in each patient determine the best procedure. For example, lesions in the inner quadrant of the breast require extended radical mastectomy, while women with very small outer quadrant tumors and negative palpable nodes may sometimes have as good a prognosis with a modified radical. In most cases, however, a Halstead radical mastectomy is the treatment of choice.

LUMPECTOMY

Recently, there has been a lot of attention paid to the procedure known as lumpectomy. If this were as effective as more extreme surgery, what a boon to women with breast cancer! Once again, though, we need to restate the goal of treatment, which is ultimately cure. The survival rates after lumpectomy have not been as good as those obtained by more extensive surgery. The main advocate of lumpectomy has been a surgeon named Dr. George Crile. Using this procedure in a poorly controlled study, he reported a ten-year survival rate of 43 percent. (The survival rate at Sloan Kettering for Stage I and Stage II patients is 82 percent.)

Crile himself has stated: "My stand on the treatment of breast cancer has been widely misunderstood. Many surgeons believe that I advocate what the British call lumpectomy and irradiation. Nothing could be farther from the truth." Crile looked for less radical surgery to treat breast cancer because he felt that women who should be treated were delaying their treatment out of fear of losing an entire breast. ". . . it is fear of this loss rather than ignorance of the significance of the lump that is the greatest cause of delay in treatment."

It would be a tragedy if women who can actually be saved by appropriate surgery are lulled by false hopes or bad statistics into choosing surgery which is not best for their condition—especially for early breast cancer, where survival rates are extremely good. Since a great many breast cancers are what is called multicentric—that is, they occur in many different places in the affected breast—simply removing one tumor may leave other areas to grow, requiring further surgery and endangering the patient's chance of cure.

AFTER SURGERY

It takes ten to fourteen days for the scar to heal, and the small drainage tubes are left in place for the first few days. The arm is swollen for a few days after surgery, especially if it was radical surgery—about 50 percent of patients experience some degree of postoperative swelling of the arm on the side surgery was performed. Pain medication can make most patients fairly comfortable.

Many hospitals now offer courses with specially trained nurses and with other women who have had mastectomies. It is very important to do certain exercises. The patient gets a little rubber ball to help exercise the hand, and this exercise helps control some of the swelling.

After the patient goes home, it is usually wise to bar visitors during the first five days. Some women are able to return to work three weeks after surgery, but there will still be some pain in the arm and it may still be swollen. Some doctors suggest that the patient stay at home and not enter stress-filled situations until she feels really better.

PROSTHESES

There are many very good kinds of artificial breasts (called prostheses) and the surgeon will suggest the best choice after the patient is sufficiently healed to wear one. An artificial breast cannot be worn immediately after surgery because the scar needs time to heal.

Breast reconstruction is a procedure very few surgeons would recommend. First, it is medically unwise because an artificial substance implanted within the breast may act as an irritant and will mask discovery of recurrence; secondly, the results just don't look that good. Reconstructed breasts do not look like or feel like natural breasts.

WHAT TREATMENT IS DONE AFTER SURGERY?

Whether or not a woman will need additional treatment after breast surgery depends to a large extent on how far the cancer has spread. For women with small tumors, no positive nodes, and no signs of distant spread, surgery will be the only treatment required. But 65 to 70 percent of patients with three or more positive nodes will have recurrence of their disease within ten years. Obviously something needs to be done with this group of patients. In the past, the major treatment for patients with positive nodes, but without distant disease, was radiation to the chest wall, armpit, and an area above the collarbone, on the side where the breast was removed. Radiation controlled the recurrence of local disease (growth of cancerous nodules) on the surface of the chest wall, in the armpit, or above the collarbone on the side of the breast cancer; however, radiation did not effect survival. Survival remained the same whether the patients were treated with radiation or not. Also, radiation did not improve the control of distant spread; patients were just as likely to get metastatic disease.

In the hope of improving survival in patients with positive nodes, various studies have been set up to evaluate the use of chemotherapy as an adjunct to surgery. *Chemotherapy* is the term used to describe treatments given to cancer patients using a chemical or a group of chemicals with the ability to interfere with cell multiplication. Several different types of cancer, not just breast cancer, respond to treatment with chemical agents. One theory of the way in which the process works is that cancer cells may be more vulnerable than normal cells to chemicals administered at certain stages of their growth, and laboratory work on animals suggests that the response is best when small amounts of tumor are present. Chemotherapy is now being employed in the adjuvant setting and the early results are very encouraging. Dr. Gianni Bonnadonna, in a randomized study, has noted a significant reduction of recurrence of cancer in patients treated with three drugs as opposed to patients treated with no drugs after radical mastectomy. His updated figures show that patients with more than four positive nodes had a 20 percent recurrence rate within three years, if they were treated with chemotherapy, while patients who were not treated with drugs had a 50 percent recurrence rate. These preliminary findings are exciting and interesting, but Bonnadonna, as well as others, cautions against overzealous enthusiasm over the preliminary results; only time will tell whether this significant difference in recurrence rate will continue and have an impact on changing survival.

If, at the time of surgery, or at some point many years after surgery, the woman is found to have metastatic disease, there are many forms of treatment that can be used, including endocrine manipulation, radiation, and/or chemotherapy. The type of treatment that is selected by a physician depends very much on how severe the disease is and what parts of the body are affected.

ENDOCRINE MANIPULATION

The aim of endocrine manipulation is to change the hormonal environment of a patient's body. For example, in premenopausal women, who are producing estrogen, the way to change the hormonal environment is to remove the source of estrogen and therefore an oophorectomy will be performed. In postmenopausal women, who are not producing estrogen, supplying them with estrogen will create this change. Some postmenopausal women have very good responses to estrogen; their cancer regresses and their appetites and sense of well-being improve. These same women may stop responding to the estrogen, in which case they are sometimes treated with androgens, which can have similar results.

One test that some hospitals consider useful in deciding whether or not to use hormone treatment is the test called estrogen binding. It is performed on tissue taken at the time of surgery. Patients with positive binding may have better response rates to the administration of estrogens or androgens. This hormonal binding ability can also be used to help solve the problem of whether a therapeutic ablation should be used (therapeutic ablation is a removal of organs such as ovaries, adrenals, or even the pituitary gland). All these organs affect the hormonal environment of the patient, and by changing hormonal environment, occasionally there can be a decrease in the amount of tumor in that particular patient. If hormonal therapy fails, the patient may then go on to chemotherapy. Whether one or more drugs are used depends again on the particular situation, because occasionally very good responses can be seen with a single chemotherapeutic agent.

In summary, breast cancer is a curable disease. Early detection is obviously very important, and if women do monthly breast exams, they may greatly improve their chances of survival. If breast cancer is discovered, then it is very important to have the appropriate surgery and follow-up. It is important to understand that even if the disease is not detected at an early stage, there are treatments available for any stage of breast cancer, and in the future, perhaps there will be new and better ones.

7

SEX AT MENOPAUSE

During and after menopause, an interesting sexual change often occurs: Women become more erotic. Some older women have more sexual fantasies, masturbate more frequently, and want sex more than when they were young. Rather than fading away with the decline of estrogen, their sexual desire increases. While this makes no evolutionary sense—why should nature have made women want sex more when they are no longer able to bear children—this phenomenon has been noted frequently, and there are several possible explanations.

One theory is based on physiology. During the menstrual cycle, there are definite hormonal changes that occur eight days out of every month, changes very similar to those which occur after menopause. During the week or so before the monthly period, progesterone and estrogen drop; the pituitary hormones show some fluctuation; but androgen, the male hormone women produce in small quantities, does not fluctuate and is unopposed by the female hormones. Androgen increases libido in both men and women, but in women its effects are usually masked by estrogen. It is easier to understand some of the physical aspects of the menopause if we realize that, in fact, we experience a "mini-menopause" every month. While some women normally experience very little variation, others notice a definitely heightened sex drive just before and during their period. Menstrual changes are unstable and last for a few days, whereas menopausal changes are more gradual and our bodies eventually adjust to them.

This chapter was written from a series of interviews with Helen Singer Kaplan, M.D., Ph. D.—Ed.

After menopause (and the great reduction in estrogen supply), our adrenal glands continue to make the same amount of androgen as before.

There are other factors which may cause an increase in sex drive. For many women, inhibitions have now worn off. This freedom from sexual taboos is an asset to the mature woman. She can enjoy sex more herself, especially now that she is freed from the burden of birth control and fear of pregnancy. She is also better able to arouse her older partner and to give him a good sexual experience, because she feels freer to use more active stimulation techniques, such as oral sex, and in general is able to show an open desire for sex. An older woman is capable of greater warmth, sensitivity, and humanity in her sexual relationships than she was as a very young woman.

CHANGES IN OUR SEXUAL ORGANS

There are some physiological changes during and after menopause which interfere with sexual response but not sexual desire. Without the stimulation of estrogen, the vagina may begin to atrophy—the tissues become thinner and more easily irritated—and may not lubricate as much. This problem can be easily corrected either by replacement therapy with oral estrogen (over which there is tremendous controversy) or by the application of topical estrogen cream (over which there is somewhat less controversy). Sometimes, Vaseline or K-Y jelly is an effective way of dealing with the problem of insufficient lubrication. But one of the best ways to prevent atrophy is to have a very regular sex life.

ATTRACTIVENESS

Women can't count any longer on youthful physical beauty and freshness to attract men, but there are other qualities that living has enhanced—the ability to express warmth and gentleness and intimacy. It is just as hard for a man as it is for a woman to find someone with whom to share an intimate relationship. For some women, self-esteem depends on the man they are able to seduce. If they are divorced, widowed, or single and can't find a man, they feel they are nothing. (The older man who needs to appeal to a good-looking teen-age girl for his own self-esteem suffers from the same problem.) Women who are now entering the menopausal period belong to a generation reared to feel that unless they can attract an attractive man, their own accomplishments and their own humanity are worthless.

One woman at sixty-nine was widowed for the fourth time. She is now happily remarried. Although not a terribly attractive woman, she is warm and sensitive and giving. Her latest husband simply adores her and is very much in love with her. She is neither rich nor beautiful so one can think of no other reason for five men wanting to marry her except that they found her so giving and warm.

If you are attractive to your partner at the age of fifty, it is not simply because you're gorgeous, but because you meet other human needs: sensitivity, intimacy, warmth. These are the assets which do not fade, but increase with age. That many personable, attractive, intelligent women have trouble finding partners should not be a source of depression or cause a loss of self-esteem to them. At middle age, the supply of available interesting men is diminished.

MAKING SEXUAL CHOICES

There are many women (some men too) who cannot enjoy sex without commitment. They become so vulnerable that if their partners do not want to continue a relationship, they experience deep depression; they are destroyed. Other women can enjoy having a casual, sensual experience even though it may not lead to a committed relationship. This is a matter of choice. If you feel that a casual encounter will lead to feelings of misery, it is not worth it.

In general, many women now in their late thirties, forties, and fifties have difficulty enjoying the new sexual freedom. Perhaps 10 percent are able to enjoy casual sex with an attractive man they have met at a party earlier that same evening. It is not so much a case of gender or biological differences as of cultural conditioning, since both younger men and younger women seem more interested in casual sexual relationships than do older women and men. Among the middle-aged and older, there seem to be few women who can enjoy sex without some emotional bond. Unfortunately, many divorced or widowed women in this group feel they must have sex in order to find a husband or get a date.

An interesting contrast to this general rule are a few women who have become sexually active very late in life, and have had positive experiences. One sixty-eight-year-old woman, who is now widowed, had never enjoyed sex in her life, yet she remained faithful to her husband. Some time after his death, she entered psychosexual therapy, feeling that she did not want to die without ever experiencing an orgasm. Her therapist taught her how to have an orgasm, and now she has a sexual relationship that she enjoys. Her relationship is not a romantic one but it does give her pleasure. It is rare for a woman to begin enjoying sex in her seventh decade, and I feel that in seeking this experience she is a courageous, marvelously spirited woman.

CHOOSING CELIBACY

Choosing to live without sexual partners is sometimes a very good alternative for women who want to have sex only with men for whom they deeply care. If celibacy is freely chosen and does not represent a constriction and a deprivation, it may be one solution. Perhaps the best way to illustrate this is to cite two case histories.

The first is a fifty-year-old woman with three children and a child by a former marriage, whose second husband left her for another woman. It was a very painful experience for her. She decided to devote herself to raising her children, and she tried to keep the family happy and going as well as possible. Having been a secretary before marriage, she took a small part-time secretarial job. She did not go out particularly often; she gave up any kind of sexuality altogether and came to a sort of peace with a very limited life. She spent most of her time with women—not out of any political belief, but because she had given up trying to meet men. This woman closed in and limited the possibilities that might enrich her life.

Another woman, forty-nine and a social worker, chose celibacy in a much different way. When she learned that her husband was dying, she said that she would never find anyone as wonderful as he. They had a truly rare relationship. After his death, she became deeply immersed in very significant women's activities. She hasn't ruled out the possibility of finding another lover, but she won't compromise on someone she does not care for deeply. Having had a wonderful relationship, she felt it was something that might happen only once in a lifetime. She is very creative and open and has started a new career related to but expanding on the one she had had.

These two women both elected celibacy, but while one is extremely constricted and limited, the other one is growing and feels marvelous and good about herself.

CHOOSING MARRIAGE

Finding another human being to share your life with can be a wonderful and exciting experience. But there are some women who just cannot bear to be alone. They do not choose marriage; they run from solitude. Often they immediately rush into a second marriage. Sometimes such a marriage works well; sometimes it is a dismal failure. In the following example, the new marriage was a success.

A woman physician lost her husband very suddenly. Within a month she was engaged and within three months she was married to another doctor, who had been recently divorced, a man quite different from her first husband. This woman's second marriage is a good one. She deeply appreciates sharing her life with someone, and she happily accommodates herself to another person, knowing that she falls apart when she feels alone.

Another woman, also terrified of being alone, was unhappily married, but would not leave her husband until she had a replacement lined up. Her second marriage was a disaster; the couple divorced within a year. She immediately married again and again was miserable. Now at forty-nine she finds herself unhappily married because she could not face being alone and cannot adjust to living with another person.

These are both women who cannot bear to be alone and immediately remarry. One woman succeeds in her new marriage because she is in touch with how much she needs to share her life and is willing to make necessary compromises. The second woman is not in touch with her need to fantasize the "perfect man," the perfect marriage. She escapes from solitude only to find that her fantasies fail her in real life.

ENRICHING YOUR SEX LIFE IN MARRIAGE

For many of us, the ideal is a one-to-one committed relationship. A few women are blessed with such a relationship for a lifetime. But partners, even in an enduring marriage, sometimes lose touch with one another; they stop communicating, and if there is one area in which communication is vital it is the area of sex. Most people have for years had secret fantasies and desires that they have never talked about to their partners. Most people don't know what their partner is experiencing; they may guess, but they don't really know and never ask. In a typical therapy session, one middle-aged man was explaining his sexual problems and complaints. The therapist intervened to ask, "Do you know what your wife feels when you make love to her?" "No," answered the husband. The therapist then asked him how long he had been married, and he responded, "Twenty-two years." During the remainder of the session, the couple simply told each other what each one felt during love-making, something they had not done in twenty-two years of marriage.

The years during which menopause occurs are also the time when good relationships become solidified and even more secure. When a woman goes through menopause and her husband does not abandon her—in fact, is closer than ever—a fantastic sense of security and peace arises; these can be the best years of a marriage. There are always some fears and insecurities, but an enduring marriage enables the couple to surmount them. The children are grown and the need to stay together for their sake no longer applies. A woman and man in such a situation can say, "It's me; it's really me; it's really us. We're still together and it still matters." This is a wonderful stage in a relationship, better than anything you could ever want in your life.

An example of this new security is illustrated in the following case: A wife was chronically depressed for twenty-five years, thinking that her husband didn't really care. Every night when he came home, she was surprised that he came home. She expected to be abandoned every day of her life. Her husband wasn't a demonstrative man but was basically very dependent on her, loved her, and was never really interested in anyone else. Around the time of her menopause, it finally dawned on her that she hadn't been rejected all these years, that her husband wanted to stay with her. A marvelous peace has settled over their marriage; they entertain together, travel together, and it's never been better. She said, "It's a different marriage; I didn't feel married until now."

CHOOSING ALTERNATIVES TO MARRIAGE

Homosexuality

Some women at the age of forty to fifty decide to become homosexual because our changing cultural attitudes now allow people who have formerly repressed their homosexuality to become more overt and to experiment more. I have known several women who were socialized to be heterosexual, were married against their impulses, and who then finally decided to do what they had always wanted and have women for lovers.

In one instance, a wealthy woman from the South, who had been raised in a very strict environment, married and had a child. Sometime later, having discovered that her husband was gay, she began to experiment and was seduced by an older woman while in her early thirties. She decided that this was the kind of relationship she wanted, and now leads a very open homosexual life-style.

Most converting to homosexuality, however, seems to be done by the time women are in their thirties. The few studies that have been made of women who are homosexuals or bisexuals have been conducted among younger women; statistics about older women exploring homosexuality as an alternative life-style do not yet exist. One woman with five grown children, who was divorced after twenty years, felt that lesbianism was the best alternative. "After fifty," she said, "it is not easy to make a new life, and there is a relief in finding yourself alone, a certain freedom from obligations. It is difficult to relearn the art of seductive flirtation and as men begin to move closer, often they just want you to cook for them, to clean for them. I found a comfortable union with another woman whose marriage also had faltered and who had been my close friend for thirty years. For us it has been a beautiful thing, not just gratification or a feeling of intimacy but real passion motivated our relationship."

Older Women, Younger Men

Some women have experimented with taking lovers much younger than themselves. For some, these affairs have been satisfying. Often, however, younger men are seeking experience and reassurance for themselves and don't really care about the older woman, except as a means to that end.

I know of two women—one a musician, the other an actress, both enormously successful in their careers—who had totally opposite experiences with younger men. The musician had been married twice before, both times to rather rigid older men. She was miserably unhappy in her marriages although her misery spurred her career; it enabled her to compose some very fine music. Today, she is living with a young man who is extremely sensitive to her emotional needs and who adores her. He is also a musician, and she seems sublimely happy. For the first time, she seems at peace, absolutely serene.

The other woman is an actress in her sixties, previously married to a physician. She led a miserable life for years and experienced an especially painful divorce. Although a very sexual, sensual woman, after her divorce she was very lonely and was involved with several unhappy relationships. One was with a young lawyer who was mainly interested in her money. They planned to go to Europe together, and she loaned him the money for the trip. When she wanted it back, he said, "Fuck you, and if you take me to court I'll say that I was your lover and that you paid me." She is now having a highly satisfying relationship with a man who is a few years younger than she is but also in his sixties.

Both women were brilliant, insightful people, but also very vulnerable. One happened to pick a sensitive, marvelous young man, and the other one picked an unscrupulous character. Sometimes older women are blinded by their vulnerability and are therefore prey to psychopathic men. There are women who say that their May/December relationships have been beautiful and totally satisfying for many years. But older women must be wary of their own insecurities and of grabbing at a "last chance," particularly if they have money.

Involved But Unmarried

Having a close relationship with a man is important to most women, but that relationship need not always lead to marriage. One woman described her feelings about such a relationship: "I, myself, am not married, but I'm very much connected to a man I care deeply for. I'd prefer marriage; he prefers our present arrangement. But because I'd rather have a connection to him than be married to eighteen other men, I've made a choice to be with him. There are advantages for me because I find that I'm extremely free to take care of my children without conflict. But there are disadvantages too. There are times when I would like him to be there, when he's halfway around the world. If I were very insecure, I would have said, 'I'm sorry I can't accept this.' But I'm secure enough to have the luxury of making this choice. He too has enough confidence to ask me to share his life in this way, knowing that he took the risk of losing me if I refused."

Women Without Partners

Living alone after being married is an enormous change and for women who feel abandoned, a painful one. If you are used to having someone there at night and in the morning, the loneliness really hurts. Women who find themselves in this situation need to learn to acknowledge and deal with this pain. The escapes—talking compulsively on the telephone, overeating, drinking too much, taking tranquilizers—don't allow one to face and deal with the situation, to say, "I really feel pain, it hurts, that's what it feels like to be alone."

What comes out of experiencing the pain is not miraculous; it's a growing sense of integration, a recognition of reality. Either you learn to live a satisfying life alone or you realize that the importance of finding another relationship outweighs the difficulty and compromise involved in finding one. It's a decision, and there is great strength to be gained in realizing one's independence, in being able to say, "I can live well alone. Look what I did this evening—I wrote a chapter (or I exercised or listened to music). I'd love to have a relationship, but I can live just fine without it."

Finding a New Partner

If you want another relationship, you probably will not succeed if you go out "hunting" obsessively for it, because if you are anxious, you'll comunicate that anxiety. The intensity of your need will scare people off. But you have to be open to the possibility of meeting someone you like. When you do meet a suitable person, you need to allow a relationship to grow. If you don't have a close relationship

SEX AT MENOPAUSE | 121

with a man you care for, you can elect to be celibate if that makes you feel good about yourself, or you can elect to try different kinds of experiences you've never had before: an affair with a younger man, a casual relationship, a relationship where you dominate, one where you allow yourself to be pursued, one where you try pursuing. These are new experiences that can teach you things about yourself that you never had the opportunity to learn.

If both partners want a good sexual experience, this is terrific. If one partner wants love and the other one wants only sex, it is a disaster, no matter what gender you are. That is why it is so wrong for psychiatrists to go to bed with their patients. Usually the patient wants love and the psychiatrist just wants to have a sexual experience. When one person wants sex and the other wants more, the situation becomes damaging—and the older woman often wants more.

For women who are divorced or single (although most would like to have an intimate one-to-one relationship), now is the opportunity to explore your sexual needs and reactions. You can elect not to go to bed with somebody if you feel like it. Or you can elect to try different situations and see what they feel like. Meet somebody, go to bed with him that night, and see how you feel the next morning. Find out how to tell a man what you like to do in bed. You are free to be adventuresome if you choose.

THE BASIC PHYSIOLOGY OF THE SEX ACT

The sexual response of both men and women seems to be one continuous curve, starting with desire and ending with a climax, but closer study reveals that for both men and women there are three *separate* phases. The first is desire; the second phase is the excitement phase (the swelling of the genitals with blood), which in the male produces erection and in the female produces swelling and lubrication of the vagina. The third phase is the orgasm, which is very similar in men and women, although it appears to be quite different. The man has two phases of orgasm. During the first, the ejaculate is squeezed into the posterior urethra located in back of the penis. This causes only a little sensation. This phase is followed a split second later by rhythmic contractions of the striated muscles at the base of the penis that expel the semen, and this is the pleasurable phase. Women's orgasms are analogous to the second phase of the male orgasm. Of course, there is no ejaculation, but stimulation around the clitoral area produces rhythmic contractions of the same type of muscles that cause ejaculation in men, and these contractions (which occur at the same rate in men and women) constitute the female orgasm.

Interestingly, there are very few gender differences in the aging process; women stop having super memories at the age of twenty-eight just as men do; women may be energetic tennis players in their twenties but by the time they are fifty they have to play doubles just the way men do. In other words, loss of memory, loss of physical stamina, skin wrinkles, varicose veins, and senility are problems for both sexes. There is one function, however, where there is a drastic difference and that is sexual function. Men, unlike women, experience a refractory period; that is, a certain amount of time must pass after an orgasm before a man can have another one. The length of this period changes dramatically with age; while an adolescent boy can have a second orgasm within another minute or 30 seconds, by the time he is fifty, he usually has to wait twelve hours. This dramatic lengthening of the refractory period is absent in women even when they are ninety-nine. Women may not always have the desire, but they have the ability. Sexual desire in the male is at its height at seventeen or eighteen and then during the twenties it gradually declines. It never disappears, but the urgency is lost somewhere around middle age. For women the reverse is true. As women grow older (unless they have physical or emotional problems) their sexual desire usually increases—even after menopause!

A woman who loves sex has a great opportunity for pleasure after menopause and should not be discouraged if she encounters a few problems caused by low estrogen levels. If she has pain on intercourse, which is caused by vaginal atrophy (thinning of the vaginal tissues), she should remember that this is something that can be remedied and should ask her doctor for help. Frequent sex will often prevent atrophy from becoming a problem.

MAKING LOVE TO AN OLDER MAN

At menopause, a woman's sexual partner or partners are usually older men. And the older man is sexually quite a different animal from what he was as an adolescent. Often he does not realize this, and the woman has not realized it either. Women do not change sexually as much as men do. If anything, they become better lovers, and more responsive. Younger women don't have orgasms as easily as younger men. Later on, men take longer and have more difficulty achieving orgasm. Happily, both partners can enjoy exciting each other, and of the three phases of sexuality—desire, excitement, and orgasm—the excitement phase continues to occur for both sexes despite aging. But orgasm in men diminishes greatly, while women stay multiply orgasmic all their lives.

The picture of the sexual male as portrayed in literature and movies is that of the adolescent male with the constant erection. Society has raised us to picture all male sexuality as adolescent male sexuality, but in reality, for most of his sexual life, a man has a different pattern of response.

By the age of fifty, a man has slower sexual responses. He doesn't have instant erections. His penis has to be played with and touched before he actually has a full erection, and it takes him longer to have an orgasm. A man may be upset and disappointed by this slowing down and may become depressed about what he feels are sexual failures. An older woman who can understand his fears is able to be helpful and patient. She can take a more active role in exciting him. (The younger woman does not have to be active with her younger lover because he just looks at her, gets an erection, and hopes that he won't come too fast.) An older man needs a good deal of actual physical stimulation. Massage parlors are attractive because the women there spend a lot of time stimulating the customers. Realizing this, a woman will apply direct tactile stimulation to her partner's penis, because he needs this before his erectile reflexes will respond. After the age of forty-five or fifty, prolonged tactile stimulation becomes very important.

Stimulation Techniques

If you are using vaseline for added lubrication, make it part of your sex play. Have your partner apply it to your clitoral area and use some to stimulate his penis, an exciting and effective way of helping a man to develop his erection.

Many older couples have begun to experiment with oral sex, and both men and women can find it immensely liberating and stimulating. Men who are slow to arouse using other techniques are often tremendously excited by oral stimulation. Some men and women, however, find the idea distasteful; obviously for them it will not be effective. But many people while in their mid-fifties and sixties begin to enjoy experimenting with new techniques; they go to erotic movies, read erotic books to one another, or experiment with a vibrator, which allows the man to give pleasure to his partner without having to be aroused and is a very reliable way for a woman to have orgasm.

IMPOTENCE IN OLDER MEN

One problem an older man may encounter is chronic physical illness, which sometimes can cause sexual problems such as lack of desire, failure to achieve orgasm, or difficulty in achieving erection.

Hormone replacement therapy is now being used for men as well as women. One needs to be extremely careful, however, for very few studies have been made of the side effects or dangers of testosterone replacement therapy. Initially there was a fear that the hormones might activate prostate cancer. At present, no conclusive studies have been reported. Before an older man with a low testosterone level is given replacement therapy, he should, of course, have a thorough physical checkup because of the possible danger of heart attacks.

Impotent men can also consider having corrective surgery. There are two kinds of procedures: One consists of an implantation of two small silicone rods, which produce a perpetual but flexible erection. The other procedure gives a man an inflatable penis. In this case, the penis is actually blown up; a small valve with a reservoir of fluid is inserted under the skin of his belly. Although this procedure is not uncomfortable for most men, about 5 percent of patients have problems with it. Most men tolerate this type of surgery well, so it is indicated if the man has sexual desire and has experienced good orgasms but is having difficulty achieving erection. In some cases, where a man has trouble having an erection, he and his partner may elect to have sex without penetration; the couple can have a very good time by mutually stimulating each other.

SEX AND FANTASY

The open use of fantasy is a marvelous aid to sexual pleasure, and sharing your fantasies with your partner can enhance lovemaking. Everybody fantasizes. We need to learn how *not* to judge our thoughts or feel foolish for having them. When people do learn to share fantasies freely, wonderful things can happen. One case history illustrates this point well: A man finally admitted to his wife what he fantasized when he made love to her—that he watched her teach a young boy to make love. The fantasy excited him and helped him function, but he had never considered telling her about it. He thought she would reject him and think the whole thing disgusting. Instead, after agreeing to try to share it, he told her, and the idea was very exciting. They began to use that fantasy in their sex play and would openly talk about it and pretend that it was happening. They began to have more erotic fun and the new delight in their sex life enhanced their whole relationship.

Many of us have to undo a lifetime of repression and fear of disclosing our sensual nature, our erotic longings. We need to learn pride and delight in ourselves as sexual beings. Fantasy and the sharing of erotic experiences, such as reading erotic books, going to erotic movies, and openly discussing one's response to them can help us be open and playful.

TOUCHING

I always advise couples who come to me for therapy that a lovely and loving way to end the day is to hug and kiss each other. Each intimate physical contact need not automatically lead to coitus. Men and women are so afraid kissing and touching must proceed to sexual intercourse that they don't touch each other. But the idea of gently touching and kissing even for five minutes before sleep is marvelous. People need to learn that it is possible to express physical intimacy and love without its having to lead to intercourse each time. One of the great deterrents to a happy sex life is performance anxiety—the woman worrying about whether she can lubricate or the man fearing he cannot produce an erection. We need to feel free to distinguish our need for sex from our longing simply to touch. If one partner does not want sex on a given occasion, it is not a rejection. It is simply an expression of individual needs and moods. Learning to be a more expressive sexual person should be a liberating and humanizing experience for us, one which frees us from the rigid gender roles, which are so very destructive to human sexuality. We need to feel that it is perfectly fine for a man to admit his vulnerability and for a woman to be active and to admit her sexual desires. The stereotyped gender roles that forbid this are residues of an oppressive upbringing; they are extremely destructive, and no sensible person really sticks to them anyway.

MASTURBATION

From infancy to old age, for men and for women, masturbation is a normal, dependable way of obtaining sexual pleasure. By now, enough studies of human sexual behavior have convinced even the most repressed and puritanical that most people masturbate—whether married or single, sexually deprived or enjoying an active sex life. Women can masturbate using their own hands—or experiment with a mechanical vibrator. Vibrators cause an intense and dependable stimulation and are used to teach women who have never experienced orgasm how to achieve one. They should be used to stimulate the clitoris. The pastel plastic phallic-shaped vibrators don't work internally, although many women mistakenly insert them into their vaginas. It is a good idea to choose a vibrator that makes as little noise as possible.

Masturbation need not always be a solitary act. Masturbating with your partner can be exciting, a way of sharing sex without putting any burden of performance on a man who has difficulty having as many orgasms as he used to. Sharing sex together at the excitement stage is very pleasurable and allows the woman to have as many orgasms as she desires. An older man may ejaculate only once a week, but he can still enjoy making love. Closeness, intimacy, sharing pleasure are far more important than whether every single encounter ends in orgasm. A case history will illustrate this point.

The case is of a couple who had not had sex for six or seven years. The man, who had a chronic disease, consulted me first because he could not have full erections. His illness was one of the physical causes of his problem. Although he could still have partial erections, he was so fearful of failure that he was afraid to express himself sexually. When his wife came to a therapy session, she expressed the feeling she had repressed for all the many years she had been struggling to deny her own sexual impulses, the feeling that he didn't desire her. He told her that he did, but that he didn't touch her for fear she would expect him to have an erection and initiate intercourse. This couple had three choices. They could continue their separate celibacy; he could have an operation, which would provide him with an erection; or they could have sex—touching and kissing and stimulating —without penetration. The husband sat quietly, considering how to respond, and the wife said quite suddenly, "Listen, I want to try fooling around." Her response delighted her husband; he saw that she didn't regard him as just a penis. They developed a pattern of sex play, which involved stroking and kissing each other whenever they wished. Sometimes one and sometimes both partners had a manual orgasm. The new level of intimacy they have achieved is a good example of the way in which the sexual revolution has affected older people. Here is a woman who is free to express her sexual needs openly and a man who is free to express his vulnerability. Together they have made a mutually satisfying adjustment to the changes of aging and they now enjoy the closest, most intimate relationship that they have ever had in all the years of their marriage.

SEX THERAPY

Sex therapy is one of the newer forms of therapy and is not everywhere available, nor is it appropriate for everyone. But where available and when indicated, it should not be considered the court of last resort; it should be the first approach that is tried with a sexual problem. If treatment is not successful (and it isn't always successful even in the best of hands) then the very process of treatment may point to other avenues of therapy. For example, just as a man starts getting erections again he may get very anxious, or a woman who has begun to feel pleasure by being touched gently may withdraw from her excitement and say, 'No, don't touch me." Both of these people may need deeper psychotherapy to deal with their anxieties.

At present, there is a limited number of sex therapy programs and of adequately trained therapists. As sex therapy becomes more integrated into medicine, more medical centers will offer a sexual program. Eventually, every psychiatric and mental health facility will have programs for treating sexual problems, but right now the demand is much greater than the supply.

Psychosexual therapy (the form of treatment I prefer) combines sexual exercises, which the couple practice in the privacy of their home, with couple therapy and examination of each individual's emotional problems. Some sexual problems are surprisingly easy to resolve, usually those arising from ignorance and simple performance anxiety. But sometimes deeper anxieties and fears come to light during therapy and require more extensive treatment.

A DIFFICULT TRANSITION

The specific sex problems caused by menopause are relatively easy to deal with. As has been pointed out earlier, the basic physiological problem that can interfere with sexual pleasure, vaginal atrophy, can be treated with topical estrogen cream or with over-the-counter preparations such as Vaseline or K-Y jelly. The difficult problems are the emotional ones, for this is a time of sexual transition. There is a crisis for a woman. Rather than being sexually passive she needs to learn how to be a more active lover. For a man, the transition is to a different view of sexuality, which emphasizes pleasure rather than performance. This is a period when both partners can be terribly vulnerable.

It is hard for a woman to be patient when she feels vulnerable, hard for her to realize that the man is very vulnerable himself, probably more so than she is. If he can't get an erection quickly, he will feel worse about it than she will, and he will avoid sex because he is so afraid of failure. The greatest assets a woman can have are her warmth, her understanding, and her strength.

If she can be sensitive to his fears and say, "I feel terrible too, look at these wrinkles," if they can be vulnerable together, they will increase their sense of intimacy, a far more important ingredient in the quality of one's sex life than sexual acrobatics and the sheer number of orgasms. If women can become more active sex partners, they can increase both their own and their lovers' enjoyment. It may be a difficult adjustment for a woman who has been accustomed to take the passive role in lovemaking and has relied on her mere physical presence as a stimulus for her partner. Now, when a man needs more direct tactile stimulation, it is important to realize that it is not because the woman is no longer attractive (unfortunately, a common interpretation), but rather because the man is no longer an adolescent.

A secure man will realize that women are also vulnerable at this time and will try to offer reassurance. He can say, "I don't get an erection right away because of my age, but I think you are wonderful, you give me pleasure, and I enjoy kissing you." This will make the woman feel valued and attractive and consequently more responsive.

DON'T FULFILL A NEGATIVE IMAGE

There is a myth that aging means growing uglier. This is a self-fulfilling prophecy. If a woman looks in the mirror and says, "Oh, my God I'm forty-eight, why bother," she's accepting a very damaging cultural assumption. Rather than say, "Oh, I'm forty pounds overweight and that has got to come off," she says, "I'm forty-eight; I'm supposed to be fat." If no one has ever told her that she will become ugly and less desirable at menopause, she can as easily become an elegant fifty-five-year-old woman, vital and attractive and interesting. As women, we need to ask ourselves: "Are we fulfilling society's negative expectations; are we sabotaging ourselves?" Our impulses to take care of our bodies, to wear clothes that make us feel good, are healthy.

By realizing this, you will continue to be a sexual human being. By treating yourself as one and by remaining interested in sex and open to new ways of expressing your sensual nature, you can make menopause a truly liberating time.

8

IS THERE A MALE MENOPAUSE?

In recent years there has been new interest in adult development and, with this, in the mid-life years. For women, this period has been associated with the menopause in most people's minds. Recently questions have been raised about the significance of the actual biological changes of the menopause in determining the mid-life crises for women. The difficulties for women seem, according to researchers, to be as much related to the loss of the family support, status, and self-esteem that come with the reproductive role as they are with the actual ending of the capacity to bear children.

For men, there is no clear-cut connection between any biological changes and mid-life crises. There are certainly physiological changes accompanying the process of growing older that have a profound influence on a man's sense of his life and his strength and that affect his self-esteem. But the dramatic event of the cessation of menses has, of course, no direct parallel. There is thus no external marker of the period of "male climacteric," and it is not accurate to consider this period "male menopause."

Yet there are developmental changes and life experiences that do combine to create a mid-life crisis for men.

MANIFESTATIONS

These have been manifested in a variety of ways. Attention has been drawn to this period by a number of social events: Studies show that divorces, extramarital affairs, sexual problems, and depression are most prominent in men between forty and sixty, and some studies place this crisis earlier. If a man remarries, the woman he chooses is often considerably younger than he.

A career change may be symptomatic. Corporations, having trained executives at some expense, have become concerned with a trend for men in their late thirties to leave and seek a second career.

Some men seek to change their life-style. Gauguin is perhaps one of the most famous examples. He left his wife, family, and a relatively staid life working in a bank to live in the South Seas and become a painter. A contemporary version of this is the man who decides to abandon the city and seek a "simpler" life in the country.

Some men develop symptoms—sometimes irritability, fatigue, restlessness, anorexia, insomnia, often indecisiveness. Depression may be perceived as hopelessness, sadness, or pessimism, or may be expressed in physical symptoms.

Sexual symptoms are a very important component, particularly impotence or fear of impaired performance. There are some sexual changes that occur with aging, which will be discussed in more detail later. They are often perceived by the individual as a loss of sexual power and ability. The process may be circular. Changes in sexual performance and interest, frequent in mid-life, can then lead a man to avoid sex, or to become anxious about his performance. Both of these usually lead to further difficulties, which may entrench the sexual problem.

Dr. Helmut J. Ruebsaat, who studies men undergoing the "male climacteric," describes a wide range of symptoms, which include urinary irregularities, fluid retention, hot flashes. cardiac symptoms, itching, and a variety of other psychosomatic problems. Many of these can be the equivalents of anxiety and depression.[1]

PRECIPITANTS

Often, the precipitant is some experience that confronts him with the finiteness of life and opportunity. There may be an illness, particularly a heart attack. Sometimes it is the heart attack of a friend or relative. Sometimes the awareness of some change in his own physical

1. Helmut J. Ruebsaat, *The Male Climacteric* (New York: Hawthorn Books, 1975).

response is enough to remind him that he is not the man he used to be. Some men respond to this gradual perception by denying that any changes are taking place, until some experience suddenly makes the denial break down. One forty-year-old lawyer had been playing basketball with friends every weekend. One Sunday he fell and ruptured a tendon. Although the injury healed well, he became depressed. He felt vulnerable. "My body would not have behaved this way ten years ago," he said. Another man at forty-five was told on a routine physical exam that he had high blood pressure. He became anxious, preoccupied with death. This was his first illness, the first time his "physical perfection" had been threatened. He felt that there was little distance between the first "chink in the armor" and the eventual disintegration of death. His masculine pride had rested in the ideal of a perfect body and this was damaged by the illness.

Awareness of aging changes constitutes a similar masculine blow. A common one is baldness. Others are gray hair, wrinkles, loss of skin tone, development of a paunch, and the need for reading glasses or bifocals. Some begin to notice small memory lapses. Other precipitants are disappointments in work: For instance, a financial reversal may set off more despair than the actual reality warrants. A missed promotion may bring acute awareness that one has slipped off the ladder of "success." Success itself, when achieved, may seem to be empty, especially compared with one's original fantasies of what it would bring. Conflicts with adolescent children, competitive feelings with younger men who seem to be emerging and challenging may be important components.

> Mr. Y is a forty-five-year-old lawyer, working for a medium-sized firm. As a young man he was interested in writing but had little time during law school and after to devote to anything but what was connected with his work. He has achieved some prominence, but recently when a committee was being formed to study a particular problem he was not chosen. His younger partner, who is interested in the same area, went instead. He is aware of feeling disappointed but not shattered. A new assignment leads to many late hours of work. He is unusually tired. He finds his interest in sex lessened, as he comes home tired and enervated. He begins to drink more; he finds that he is unable to sustain an

erection. The few times he does attempt intercourse his wife seems to withdraw as well. More drinking leads to further difficulties. His twenty-year-old son fails his college math course. A young secretary, who has just come to work, clearly indicates that she thinks of him as an "older" man and not interesting. A colleague close to him in age has a mild heart attack. Mr. Y becomes very depressed. He feels that life is soon to end, that he will never realize his dream of writing, and that even his successful work is unrecognized. He drinks further, accentuating his sexual difficulties without being aware of the cause. His sexual life is failing, and his family is disappointing him.

Another man, forty-eight, is a businessman, manufacturing chemicals. He has moved with his family three times—to various urban centers, each time enlarging his business, changing the products slightly. Each time he achieves moderate success, but is not able to find real friendships among his associates or stability in the growth of the company. He wonders whether he has missed something by pursuing this kind of work. His children, with whom he spent much time, grow into adolescence and begin to leave home. His wife becomes active in the community and acquires a name for herself as a civic leader. She then obtains a rewarding and demanding job. He is not aware of feeling depressed, but begins to want to leave the business and the city and move west, to a rural area, and try specialized farming, feeling that opportunities are declining in the city, pollution is rising, and there will soon be no future for American cities. How can one understand these changes?

All people continue in their development as they grow older. Erikson describes life as a cycle, with developmental stages characterizing individuals from infancy through old age.[2] However, data on the details of adult life stages have been sparse. Recently, a research group at Yale led by psychologist Daniel Levinson has conducted a study of stages in the adult lives of men.[3] They have done intensive inter-

---

2. Erik Erikson, *Childhood and Society* (New York: W. W. Norton, 1964).
3. D. J. Levinson, C. M. Darrow, et al., "The Psychosocial Development of Men in Early Adulthood and Mid-Life," in *Life History Research Psychopathology*, vol. 3, ed. D. F. Ricks (Minneapolis, Minn.: University of Minnesota Press, 1974).

views with a carefully selected group of forty men. Ten are executives, ten are blue- and white-collar workers, ten are writers, and ten are biologists at different stages of their careers. Dr. Levinson categorizes the developmental periods of adulthood into a series of stages: early adulthood, twenty–forty; middle adulthood, forty–sixty; late adulthood, sixty plus. He further conceptualizes several periods "within which a variety of biological, psychodynamic, cultural, social, structural, and other timetables operate in only partial synchronization." They are:

(1) Leaving the family—from high school to twenty–twenty-four.

(2) Getting into the adult world—when the center of gravity shifts from the family of origin to a new home base. This is roughly from the early twenties to twenty-seven or twenty-nine, a time of exploration and initial choice—establishing an occupation, adult friendships, an initial life structure. An important component of this period is the dream with which many men enter adulthood.

(3) The settling down period ordinarily begins in the early thirties—with deeper commitments, pursuit of more long-range plans and goals. The aspect of "making it," attaining goals, becomes important. Dr. Levinson points out that parts of the self are inevitably left out or remain dormant in the pursuit of other goals. The peak of this settling down period is the phase of:

(4) becoming one's own man, in the late thirties. This is accompanied by the man's "feeling that no matter what he has accomplished to date, he is not sufficiently his own man." A mentor, a role that Dr. Levinson describes as important in adult development, is given up by forty. This is also the stage of Erikson's "generativity versus stagnation," where caring for adults and taking responsibility in the adult world is important.

(5) the mid-life transition is next, in which the central issue is the disparity between what has been gained and what an individual wants for himself.

(6) Somewhere around age forty-five restabilization takes place in which a new life structure begins to take shape and provide a basis for living in middle adulthood.

Dr. Levinson describes a period that he calls the mid-life transition which reaches its peak some time in the early forties and then undergoes a period of restabilization in the middle forties, settling into middle adulthood around age forty-five. This is a developmental phase

—between the establishment of one's adult self and later adulthood. "A developmental transition," he says, "is a turning point . . . [which] may go smoothly or may involve considerable turmoil. The mid-life transition occurs whether the individual succeeds or fails in his search for affirmation by society." He points out that a transition is inevitable—the character and form of it varies.

This emphasizes the essential normality of transitions, and even crisis points, in a person's life. At any transition point there is both 'possibility for developmental advance and of great threat to one's self." Dr. Levinson points out that "men such as Freud, Jung, Eugene O'Neill, Frank Lloyd Wright, Goya, and Gandhi went through a profound crisis around forty and made themselves creative geniuses through it." Others, such as Dylan Thomas and Sinclair Lewis, could not manage this crisis and destroyed themselves in it. He also stresses that men who do not make changes at all in the course of their lives become terribly weighted down and lose the vitality one needs to keep developing.

This view of a crisis as a time of increased potential is an important one. There are analogous periods for women—and at other times of life. For instance, adolescence and pregnancy are times for women when many potential developmental pathways are opened and the possibility for growth as well as the possibility for regression exists. These periods, then, can be regarded as a crossroads, when "new personality growth is possible and some degree of personality change inevitable." It is clearly a time of confrontation and assessment.

What are the major issues with which a man is dealing in this period? One is the awareness of the finiteness of life. The knowledge that one will some day die is very difficult to deal with psychologically. Bodily decline and mortality have been alluded to above.

The measure of achievement is particularly poignant in relation to one's sense of the limitedness of life. In this culture, self-esteem for men is strongly connected with achievement and performance. The relationship of mid-life depression to this is pointed out by Margaret Mead: "It's a question of the order of achievement, and the way it paces biological change. . . . In our society, depression comes when men realize that they've achieved all they're going to achieve."[4] In other cultures this may be different. Sol Worth, co-author of *Through*

---

4. Quoted in Martha Weinman Lear, "Is There a Male Menopause?" *New York Times Magazine*, 28 January 1973.

Navaho Eyes, says, "At age forty-five when all most of us have to look forward to is getting knocked off, the Navaho is stepping into a new hierarchy. Now he is a leader. He doesn't have to perform. . . . He does other things better, like giving advice and orders. If we're talking about climacteric depression as a biocultural event, it doesn't appear to exist here."[5]

In our culture, achievement is strongly connected with masculinity. Masculinity has rested on a number of qualities, and criteria have varied with an individual's social class, cultural group, and family patterns. However, the central components have been strength, activity, aggressiveness, competence, effectiveness, and sexual potency. A man's self-esteem has been closely connected with his masculinity, and this is challenged in the mid-life period.

The changes of this period have been described as if they are primarily related to the effect of the confrontation with limits, losses, endings.

It is important to consider also the genuine development and growth that takes place. Dr. Levinson (in an article for *McCall's*[6]) describes the changes for a man which occur in his images of women. When he marries, as a young man, his "dominant feminine image is related to the ideal of the mother" and he unconsciously chooses a wife with that in mind or projects those feelings and fantasies onto the woman he marries. As he grows into middle age, he may genuinely want another feminine image—less a mother and more a peer and lover. He has also by then usually had children and experienced the maternal image of his wife via some identification with his children. If the relationship with his wife has not changed, he may experience her as the negative mother who holds him back from realizing himself.

There are personality changes as well. Dr. Bernice Neugarten, in her and her students' many studies of mid-life, stresses the importance of introspection, contemplation, and reflection in middle age.[7] This is also a time, she has found, when people are in a position of "command," of authority, of "prime." It is the fleeting nature of this period that forms part of the crisis.

---

5. Sol Worth and John Adair, *Through Navaho Eyes* (Bloomington, Ind.: Indiana University Press).
6. Maggie Scarf, "Husbands in Crisis," *McCall's*, June 1972.
7. Bernice Neugarten, ed., *Middle Age and Aging* (Chicago: University of Chicago Press, 1968).

SEXUAL CHANGES—AGE OF ONSET

Let us take a closer look at some of the physical changes that do occur. Sexual functioning does change with increasing age. For men, normal sexual response consists of a period of arousal or excitement marked by penile erection, which lasts for a variable time until the orgasmic or ejaculatory phase. Then there is a resolution phase, during which the penis returns to a flaccid state. There is then a refractory period—the time during which an individual is unable to have another erection. With aging, there are some definite changes. The reaction time for the penis to reach full erection increases. "It is at least doubled and frequently trebled as the individual male passes through his fifties and into the sixty- and seventy-year age status."[8] Once achieved, erection may be maintained for longer periods of time without ejaculation. This ability is associated with the aging process. The younger man who develops a full penile erection may partially lose it and then regain it several times during any sexual cycle. For the older man, this is increasingly difficult. Once an erection is lost without ejaculation, may older men experience difficulty regaining it, regardless of the continuation of sexual stimulation that was previously effective. With aging, there are fewer orgasmic contractions. The refractory period lasts for an increased time as the man ages, and the resolution stage is much faster.

Although sexual responsiveness and interest gradually diminish with age for men, this is highly individual. The most important determinant in the ability to maintain sexual functioning is consistency of active sexual expression. Secondary impotence, i.e., impotence in someone previously potent, does increase sharply after the age of fifty, but Masters and Johnson have found this treatable in a high percentage of cases.

Masters and Johnson found that there are six factors that contribute to the involution of male sexual responsiveness. These are (1) monotony or boredom, (2) preoccupation with career or economic pursuits, (3) mental or physical fatigue, (4) overindulgence in food or drink, (5) physical or mental infirmities of either the man or his partner, and (6) fear of performance, influenced by any of the factors above. They

---

8. William H. Masters, and Virginia E. Johnson, *Human Sexual Response* (Boston: Little, Brown, 1966).

feel strongly about the reversibility of secondary impotence, stating that "the fallacy that secondary impotence is to be expected as the male ages is probably more fully entrenched in our culture than any other misapprehension. While it is true that the aging process, with associated physical involution, can reduce penile erective adequacy, it is also true that the secondary impotence is in no sense the inevitable result of the aging process. . . . In addition, . . . most secondary impotence associated with the aging process can be transitory in character. In most instances, secondary impotence is a reversible process for all men regardless of age unless there is a background of specific surgery or physical trauma."[9]

Adaptations to changing sexual functioning can be made if the man does not feel too threatened. Actually, some men who have had difficulty with premature ejaculations have an easier time as they get older. It is also possible to learn new techniques. It is important to shift from sexual "performance" as an orientation to a goal of mutual sexual experience.

Anxiety about sexual performance, diminished satisfaction with women, disappointment in a marriage have led to an increase in the divorce rate among couples married twenty to twenty-five years. Some men look for new sexual partners to reassure themselves about their virility and continued attractiveness, or to pursue again fantasies of ideal women, which had been given up when they married, or to find in the new marriage a source of excitement absent in other areas of his life.

Dr. Helmut J. Ruebsaat points out that some middle-aged men "experience a revival of long-dormant homosexual interest"[10] in part in response to these same issues. This may leave the woman feeling particularly angry and excluded, since she feels she cannot compete at this level.

The emphasis in our culture on youth and youthfulness makes for difficulties for an aging person. Jobs are less available, women may find him less attractive, the normal changes of aging such as graying hair or baldness, which in some societal contexts command the respect due to wisdom and experience, are considered shameful and necessary to hide. For men it is nevertheless easier than for women, whom society penalizes even more severely when they no longer look young.

9. Ibid., p. 203.
10. Ruebsaat, *The Male Climacteric.*

FAMILY

The family context is important as well.

Although a man's self-definition rests more on occupation and less on relationships with others than does that of a woman, the importance of family members in providing emotional nurture and care and filling out his life is considerable. The middle-aged man is usually the father of teen-age children, striving for their own independence and moving out of the family. His dreams for them, part of his own-self image, come up against reality and sometimes disappointment. The loss of their actual presence and the changes in the character of the relationship are also important.

As with attitudes toward the menopause in women, the attitudes toward what sociologists term "postparental life" seem to vary with class. Upper-middle-class people have an appreciably more favorable outlook on the postparental period than lower-middle-class people.

AGE

The age of this mid-life crisis is also not agreed upon. Since there are probably differences in the experience that is referred to as the mid-life crisis, the age varies. Levinson thinks this stage reaches its peak in the early forties, others see it as later. Cultural, class, and ethnic factors undoubtedly play a role, since these influence expectations and self-perception. Bernice Neugarten, in her studies of middle age, feels it comes later to the better educated, since middle-class men usually delay having children. The degree to which a man's self-esteem is dependent on physical strength, sexual performance, youthful appearance, and other attributes that characterize early adulthood, rather than those values attained after some work, such as professional success or wisdom, certainly affects his sense of peak—and of waning—powers. The loss of parents is also important in bringing on the awareness of being the dominant and older generation.

For some men, the mid-thirties is the critical time. One study describes Henry VIII's divorce of Catherine of Aragon when he was disappointed at having no male heir, and his subsequent many marriages, as a mid-life crisis in a narcissistic and vulnerable man.[11]

11. Miles Shore, "Henry VIII and the Crisis of Generativity," *Journal of Interdisciplinary History*, vol. 2, no. 4, Spring 1972, p. 16.

As men and women age, important differences exist. Bernice Neugarten describes changes in men in the direction of greater affiliative and nurturant responses. That is, they move in a "feminine" direction, while women may become less guilty about their aggressive and egocentric impulses.[12]

Dr. Levinson also describes an emergence and integration of the more feminine aspects of the self as more possible at mid-life for men, in contrast to the "masculinity" predominant in the "settling-down" period preceding it.[13]

MEN AND WOMEN

This brings up an important issue in the relationship between men and women in the mid-life period. The developmental timetable and the integration of needs and responses may be quite different for each.

For men, the relationship to work is crucial in the definition of self and evaluation of accomplishments. This is established at varying ages in various occupations but has occurred by middle age. For women, often occupied in their twenties and thirties with children, the forties have marked the beginning of a second phase—and a return to school or work. For the man in the reevaluation of the thirties or forties, the assessment of the guiding dream, in Levinson's terms, and the attainment or disappointment of this fantasy can be a major issue in the crisis. For the woman the conceptualization of her life in terms of the fulfillment of *her* dream is rare. Most women seek fulfillment via their relationships to others. The freedom to pursue one's own dream is often more difficult, and often becomes a possibility only after children are older. This may change in the current social climate of support for women's career commitments, but it has not yet changed for the majority of women. The phase of her increased exploration of and investment in the world outside the family may coincide with transition in a very different direction for her husband.

By and large women have maintained greater interpersonal networks of support and friendship than have men. Jesse Bernard, a sociologist

12. Bernice Neugarten, "Adult Personality: Toward a Psychology of the Life Cycle," *Middle Age and Aging* (Chicago: University of Chicago Press, 1968).
13. Levinson, Darrow, et al.

(author of *The Future of Marriage*), points out that with the widespread move of women into work, these friendships and support networks have been destroyed. Women turn to their husbands for support. Men often are not able to provide this, not having been trained to be expressive.[14]

The mid-life period for women can be seen as both a period of adaptation to separations and losses and a period when new energy is released for creative activity—energy that had been previously focused on family needs. The exits of children are ambivalently regarded—but one or another view predominates. In a family that experiences the leaving of children as a beginning for them and actually an extension of family supports, the women is more likely to feel the creative expansion of the mid-life years. Where children's exits are only separations and desertions, the family feels smaller, and support is withdrawn.[15]

Another potential disparity is seen in sexual relationships. Women's sexual interest and performance peaks at a later age than men's. Although this may be more cultural than biological, it is a widespread experience. Gynecologists report that many more couples are coming for sexual counseling and that the impetus is often from the woman.

Sexuality has different meaning for different people, varying also with the periods in their lives. For women, self-esteem has been associated with feeling feminine, and for many women this involves feeling attractive and desirable. Women who experience illness or mutilative surgery such as mastectomy or hysterectomy are concerned about their husbands' or lovers' response to their bodies and often experience sexual interest as reassuring and an affirmation of their worthwhileness.

The effects of aging can be experienced as damaging to self-esteem, since youthful attractiveness is so highly valued. A husband's concern with potency and performance may come at precisely the wrong time for his wife, who herself has greater sexual needs and also may be in need of reassurance about her importance to him and about her capacity to arouse interest and affection.

She may be vulnerable to the competitive and provocative behavior

14. Jesse Bernard, *The Future of Marriage* (New York: Bantam, 1973).
15. Joan Zilbach, "Family Aspects of the Mid-Life Phase" (presented at the annual meeting of the American Psychiatric Association, 1975).

of adolescent daughters—or sons. Sometimes the awareness of their children's sexuality causes the parents anxiety, and sexual problems may emerge.

If her husband is at loose ends, depressed, symptomatic, when a woman needs support from him or is looking for a renewed relationship once children are less involving, she may become angry—often unconsciously. This leads to further distance and loneliness for both, with recriminations and counteraccusations.

Sometimes the mid-life crisis for a man appears with considerable turmoil. His wife may respond to it as if it were an illness, an alien presence, rather than a developmental experience. If he blames the marriage for his disappointment with his life, her guilt at having failed may lead her to accept this externalization. Her anger may lead her to shift the blame to him—and the alienation leads to an impasse.

What can be done if there are problems? Understanding and recognition of the feelings are very important. Dr. Ruebsaat describes the relief he felt to have some awareness of what was happening to him—and to have a name for it and know it was happening to others.

Sometimes a crisis such as the discovery of an affair, or fantasies about one, can lead to new honesty about a relationship. Allowing and encouraging a husband to talk about his feelings about his marriage can be very helpful—although painful. Tolerating another person's depression or despair is difficult but important.

SEXUAL THERAPY

If there are sexual problems, professional help should be considered. Newer techniques of sexual counseling, as well as psychotherapy—for the couple, family, or individual—can be evaluated.

The "new" sex therapies involve specific treatment procedures for specific dysfunctional syndromes. Usually both partners are involved, since the interaction between them is seen as the problem and both are assumed to be contributing. The treatment depends for success on a sense of security and trust, and relief of excessive judgment, criticism, need for control, guilt, and anxiety about performance.

Sometimes the therapist suggests a period of coital abstinence to reduce performance anxiety and facilitate communication. There is erotic stimulation but no pressure to perform, so confidence gradually builds.

Marital therapy or counseling focuses on the interaction between the partners. Clarification and understanding of each person's patterns of relating to the other, as well as expectations and needs brought to the relationship from early life, coupled with current experiences, makes it possible for both to change, air feelings, confront disappointment, abandon old responses, and arrive at more appropriate new ones. It also sometimes provides a setting where both can talk to each other and learn about the other's feelings in an environment where the presence of the therapist prevents a recurrent argument from repeating itself.

What about hormone treatment? Even if male mid-life crisis symptoms are not caused by hormone deficiencies, is there anything to be gained by using them therapeutically? Some feel that there is. When given testosterone replacement therapy (testosterone is an androgen, a male sex hormone), some men do show an improvement in depression and sexual functioning. Others report no benefit from replacement therapy. Testosterone in the normal person is an essential contribution to sex drive in both men and women. The long-term effects of increased doses of testosterone over a long period of time is not yet known.

More traditional psychotherapy may be indicated if either person is very depressed or upset, or if the issues stirred up are lifelong problems stemming from unresolved relationships and feelings. For a woman, psychotherapy or counseling may be helpful in sorting out her own reactions. Men are sometimes more reluctant to accept help —even in the face of suffering.

Psychotherapy does not have to be intensive or long to be effective. Sometimes crisis-oriented treatment offers important help with a given problem. It can also help to turn a disruptive period into a developmental and maturing one.

For a woman to come to terms with her own expectations of her life and with the realities of her husband's dilemmas and distress can also be a significant contribution to her own development.

9

HELPING NATURE: DIET, EXERCISE, AND COSMETIC SURGERY

In 1923, the U.S. National Center for Health Statistics reported that the average woman's life span was 58.5 years; by 1974 the figure had risen to an all-time high of 75.8! If you are experiencing your menopause now, you have a further life expectancy of almost thirty years. What will those years bring? For many women, the whole idea of growing older is fraught with fears of illness and social uselessness, yet it need not be so.

In his study of longevity, Dr. Alexander Leaf of Harvard found an interesting factor that correlated with long life in three widely different geographical areas. Among the peoples of the Caucasus mountains, among the Hunza in Kashmir, and among the natives of the Andean valley in Ecuador, centenarians were ten to twenty times as frequent as in the populations of the United States. Some people of these three different cultures lived to 130 or more. Even more amazing was the discovery that they were still active both physically and mentally. Retirement was unknown. These people continued to lead useful lives, some even continuing to farm at the age of 110. Dr. Leaf found that there were certain habits and values common to these three very different cultures: respect for the elderly, enjoyment of life and work, low-calorie diets (about two-thirds of our own intake), the married state, some moderate consumption of alcoholic beverages, and above all *great physical activity* throughout life. It is possible that these people have some genetic predisposition toward a long life, but even though longevity may be determined partly by our heredity, the manner in which we lead our lives is the most important factor.

HEALTH DECISIONS AT MENOPAUSE

You stand, at menopause, on the threshold of half of your adult life. There are as many years ahead as you have left behind. What will the quality of those years be? It is within your power to make decisions that foster health, vitality, and attractiveness.

Do you smoke? Smoking is correlated with an increased risk of heart attacks and has been shown to lead to lung cancer and emphysema. Interestingly, some of the damage done to lungs *before* disease sets in is reversible if you do stop smoking. Cigarettes are a major health hazard, and your decision to give up smoking could add immeasurably to your health and vitality. Also to your attractiveness. Dermatologists and plastic surgeons have known for years that smoking promotes wrinkling of the skin about the mouth and eyes.

Do you drink? Alcohol in moderation is fine. A general guideline would be somewhere under three ounces of eighty-proof liquor a day. Large amounts of liquor can cause liver damage and can lead to vitamin deficiencies.

Do you weigh too much? Overweight, like smoking and drinking, puts you at higher risk for a variety of conditions: for example, heart disease, diabetes, and certain types of cancer. About 1,500 to 2,000 calories per day, or about 14 calories per pound of body weight, are needed for a *moderately active* woman to maintain her normal weight. To lose weight one must cut down on calories and/or increase physical activity to speed up the burning of calories.

WEIGHT

In general, you should now weigh about what you did weigh (or *should* have weighed) at age twenty. But as we grow older our body form continues to change, and especially around the time of menopause we notice a redistribution of weight. Even if a woman weighed at fifty what she weighed thirty years before, her waistline would be larger, her stomach rounder, and the middle portion of her body generally thicker. The precise cause for this change in weight distribution is not known. It is not likely that it is simply a lack of estrogen, since the process begins in the thirties when estrogen is high. Perhaps some of it may be due to the effect of gravity over the years or the aging of musculature and bones. To a certain extent, this tendency

146 | THE MENOPAUSE BOOK

can be counteracted by exercise and constant attention to posture. In itself, it is not a problem of overweight nor is it a reason to give up the goal of having a trim, well-cared-for body.

The following chart will guide you easily enough:

DESIRABLE WEIGHTS
Women of Ages 25 and Over
Weight in Pounds According to Frame (In Indoor Clothing)

HEIGHT (with shoes on) 2-inch heels		SMALL FRAME	MEDIUM FRAME	LARGE FRAME
Feet	Inches			
4	10	92– 98	96–107	104–119
4	11	94–101	98–110	106–122
5	0	96–104	101–113	109–125
5	1	99–107	104–116	112–128
5	2	102–110	107–119	115–131
5	3	105–113	110–122	118–134
5	4	108–116	113–126	121–138
5	5	111–119	116–130	125–142
5	6	114–123	120–135	129–146
5	7	118–127	124–139	133–150
5	8	122–131	128–143	137–154
5	9	126–135	132–147	141–158
5	10	130–140	136–151	145–163
5	11	134–144	140–155	149–168
6	0	138–148	144–159	153–173

Courtesy of Metropolitan Life Insurance Company

CHANGES IN CALORIE NEEDS

Not so many years ago weight charts showed that people got heavier and heavier as they grew older. And to many, this was entirely normal and to be expected. Today our outlook has changed entirely with the realization that "normal" is by no means the same as "desirable." What are the basic facts needed to understand this tendency to gain?

The food you ate as a child served three main purposes: (1) to create new growth in enormous quantities and to replace tissue lost through injury or weight loss, (2) to produce energy for heat and motion, and (3) to supply material for conversion into body fat as a storehouse of calories in sickness. The baby and the growing girl need many calories for *all* of these processes to serve a fast-growing, extremely active body.

After this first, rapid period of growth, you slowed down and stopped at about the age of twenty, so that fewer calories were needed for that purpose. Gradually, but probably more and more, you became less active. Therefore, fewer calories were needed for conversion into heat and motion. Clearly, if you kept on eating as much as you did when you were younger, the calories not needed for growth, heat, and motion were converted into *fat*. To remain slender, you had to take in fewer calories and stay reasonably active. Easy to say, hard to do, as so many know! Sometimes women who saw that they were getting genuinely pudgy would consult weight charts only to find that they were within an acceptable range.

These early and outmoded charts uncritically recorded regular increases of weight with age, and many people kept on eating as much as they had at a younger age even though they needed much less nourishment. By about age forty-five, a woman's rate of metabolism has slowed down. She now needs only about two-thirds as many calories as previously to *maintain* her weight. When she reaches menopause she will experience a further decrease in her caloric needs: the 10 to 15 percent her body used to maintain an active reproductive system. There is absolutely no mystery here as to why a woman gains weight at this time. She must readjust her appetite to a new level, and that adjustment is sometimes difficult.

SPECIAL PROBLEMS

As part of your general physical examination, you should discuss with your doctor any questions you have about diet in general or a reducing diet in particular. Some special dietary problems exist for women at menopause and after.

The overabundance of salt in the average diet can create problems. A moderately low salt diet contains half a gram of sodium a day. If a diet contains more than two grams of salt (sodium chloride), it is too high. The sodium in salt causes retention of extra fluid in all the body tissues and increases the blood volume, thereby increasing blood pressure.

A high cholesterol diet—rich in meat fats, cream, butter, and eggs—increases the possibility of heart disease and hastens arteriosclerosis. Certainly at menopause and ideally beginning *in childhood* we should curtail the onset of the effects of aging by eating less of these foods.

Hormone therapy can affect your diet. Women on estrogen replacement therapy may overeat in the same way that pregnant women do. In addition, estrogen increases water retention, and thus body weight. You may need to count calories more carefully if you are taking estrogens.

OSTEOPOROSIS

With the decrease in estrogen production after menopause, bones may grow lighter, thinner, and more fragile. They break more easily and bend to produce the curved spine and postural stoop of age.

To help maintain healthy bones, a diet high in calcium (a gram a day) and Vitamin D (400-500 units a day) is necessary. The high calcium intake can be achieved with skimmed milk and cheese (one eight-ounce glass of skim milk and two ounces of cheese) or with calcium tablets (four 250 mg tablets). Do not take more Vitamin D in the mistaken belief that if some is good, more is better. Too much Vitamin D can be highly toxic and therefore dangerous.

Another way to keep bones healthy is to exercise. Inactivity causes them to lose calcium and minerals. For example, during the first space flights, healthy young astronauts showed loss of calcium in their heel bones after a few days of space flight without exercise. Now all space flight personnel routinely exercise to prevent this.

VITAMIN B COMPLEX

It is a good idea to supplement your diet with one Vitamin B-complex tablet a day. This group of vitamins aids the liver in detoxifying and eliminating many chemicals—among them the pituitary hormone that may cause hot flashes. While B-complex by itself will not eliminate hot flashes, it is useful in controlling them to some extent in women who cannot or do not wish to take estrogen for this purpose.

HOW TO CHOOSE A DIET

Face the facts—maintaining or losing weight is usually difficult but worth the effort. The rewards are great: improved appearance, greater vitality, a longer life-span.

Like almost every other doctor who helps people to lose weight, I've come to realize that for many people the process is frustrating and fraught with obstacles. One thing you need is a definite plan.

Five Tips before You Begin:

1. Get a reliable scale. Knowing how you are doing is of great psychological value. Weigh yourself daily before you get dressed or eat breakfast.
2. Be prepared for plateau periods. You will not lose weight every day and may even gain at times because of fluid retention.
3. Decide on your goal using the weight/age chart or in consultation with your doctor. Determine what you want to weigh eventually. Get satisfaction from *each pound lost*. A pound or two per week is a reasonable rate, for most people. At that rate, you can lose 50 to 100 pounds a year!
4. Shop and cook with your calorie allowance in mind. Avoid recipes that call for large amounts of fat, sugar, and salt.
5. Be prepared to develop new habits of eating. The most important part of a good diet is the reeducation of your appetite and patterns of eating.

EMOTIONAL FACTORS IN REDUCING

Feelings of emptiness and deprivation are what make the most trouble for the would-be dieter. Denying yourself food can be depressing. Any time that you feel depressed, bored, lonesome, or feel that the world is treating you badly, you'll probably notice that you experience a great temptation to eat. Pay attention to these feelings in other ways: a little "gift" to yourself, a short period of leisure or amusement, something that pleases you particularly, yes, by all means —but no food.

Some hungry dieters are tempted to eat special "diet" tablets, biscuits, or cookies that contain agar or methyl cellulose. These substances swell in the stomach when taken with water, providing a sensation of fullness by distention. Since the full effects of these "fillers" are not generally understood, they are best avoided. A cup of tea or coffee (with artificial sweetener and skim milk) or diet soda may help temporarily.

FINDING THE RIGHT DIET

What's the right reducing plan for you? There are a number of good reducing diets and an even greater number of bad ones. The latest fads in diets might be the worst thing for your health.

The next section will review some of the current diet plans and theories to help you choose the best plan for you based on your knowledge of your own behavior patterns and emotional preferences.

The Group Approach

Organized weight loss plans such as Weight Watchers are often a good choice if you find it very hard to make a plan of your own and stick to it. They supply supervision, give you a schedule to follow, and instruct you in the basics of weight loss and diet cookery. For some people, the social atmosphere is helpful. If the loneliness of dieting depresses you, this may be the very thing. Group diet plans do carry a price tag, though, in terms of both money and time. Health farms, "milk farms," and spas, if well supervised medically, fall into the group diet category. They are a definite luxury for most dieters, and the most you can expect after the usual one- to two-week stay is a kind of boot in the right direction. You will still have the work of dieting to do. Think of a trip to a health spa as a marvelous luxury and an opportunity to focus on self-improvement.

Ayds

Essentially, Ayds is a sort of candy that is to be eaten before meals, with the object of lessening appetite. Some dieters do indeed find that a candy or cooky, although it is richly caloric, reduces appetite enough so that their overall calorie intake is lessened. The magic ingredient in the Ayds type of plan, however is the diet recommended in an accompanying leaflet. This diet, if followed, will produce weight loss with or without the candy. If you like the candy plan, buy your sweets for much less money and follow one of the sensible diets recommended!

Behavior Modification

Recently, we have all been hearing a lot about this method, which is based on a learning principle with a long history. The aim of behavior modification is to establish *new* responses to familiar stimuli. In the case of the would-be dieter, the familiar stimulus is hunger. The usual and undesirable response of overweight people is to eat fattening foods or larger quantities than are needed. The desired new response would be either to choose not to eat or to eat less or to eat selected, less fattening foods.

For overweight people, eating fattening foods is rewarding. Therefore, the behavior modifiers look for ways to make fattening foods seem unrewarding—and dieting the more gratifying choice. In back of this technique is that familar old principle of learning: We tend to repeat what is satisfactory and stop doing what is unsatisfactory.

Behavior modification in the laboratory is mechanical and obvious. Even a hungry rat can be taught to avoid its favorite food if he gets a shock every time he approaches it. An alcoholic may be taught to dislike whisky if he takes Antabuse, which induces extreme nausea when combined with alcohol. Such measures, however, are far too extreme for most overweight people.

In working with women who are trying to reduce we often suggest that they work out their own behavior modification programs. For example, one woman was counseled to think about her overeating in the following way: "Think pastry, potatoes, gravy—delicious—things you want to eat! But concentrate on what those foods will do to you. Think about looking unattractive in your clothes, getting tired from just a little exertion, what the extra weight does to arthritis. Now think about *not* eating those things. That means wearing a smaller size, looking good in a bathing suit, feeling sexier, living longer, feeling better. Visualize yourself getting on the scale and seeing that you've lost half a pound!"

Dieters often find that *concrete* visual imagery is a wonderful aid in putting behavior modification to work. For example, *see* yourself sitting down at the table and thinking, "I am determined not to eat so much, and I won't. That food isn't really attractive, when I think of what it will do to me! I don't really want the dessert." See yourself getting on the scale, see that rewarding number come up.

"Yes," one patient said, "but aren't you really just fooling yourself?"

Right, but it works! By all means try it.

Since the choice not to eat is such a difficult one, don't try to make it. Instead, have on hand some foods you can eat—carrot sticks already cleaned and ready to nibble, fruit, tea, or coffee. The substitute response works wonders.

The Atkins "Diet Revolution"

Dr. Robert C. Atkins's 'diet revolution" prescribes a high-fat, low-carbohydrate regime. *Theoretically,* the high fat content induces a state of acidosis, which decreases appetite by providing subliminal nausea. This is a dangerous state for anyone to be in. Such a diet induces high blood cholesterol, hastening arteriosclerosis and, thus, heart disease. In addition, it is highly dangerous for diabetics and those disposed to diabetes.

The permanence of weight loss on the Atkins diet is open to question. Acidosis causes the body to become dehydrated; weight loss that is mainly due to lower water content of the tissues is quickly restored by drinking back the water. The Atkins diet has been rejected by the National Academy of Science, the National Institute of Health, and the American Medical Association.

Eight Glasses of Water a Day

Dr. Irwin Stillman, another well-known diet doctor, recommends drinking a vast amount of water daily—at least eight glasses. While the resulting sense of fullness might help you to resist overeating, one unfortunate paradox occurs. By drinking so much water you are actually causing dehydration, which again gives the false encouragement of lost weight. The loss is largely fluid, quickly restored by drinking.

Fasting

Not eating at all is one way to lose weight rapidly, but any sudden, extreme change of diet is unwise for women forty and older. The emphasis on noncaloric fluids and vitamin pills leads to lowered blood sugar, the effects of which could cause liver damage. Proteins are lost and not replaced while fasting—and the possiblity of severe protein deficiency is a real threat.

There are No Miracle Methods

Diet fads over the years have ranged from the ridiculous to the outright dangerous. Samples of ridiculous diets once seriously proclaimed are the whipped cream diet, the lamb chop plus pineapple diet, the grapefruit diet, and other single food spectaculars.

Other diets have had very unfortunate results for their devotees. One woman following the diet regime known as "vegan" (nuts, grains, no milk, no eggs, no dairy products, no meat) became so run-down that blood poisoning resulting from a minor sore, developed into septicemia, and nearly cost her her life. However, a well-planned vegetarian diet should contain enough protein. Well-balanced vegetarian diets are healthful because they are low in calories, fat, and cholesterol content.

The danger with so many of the so-called miracle diets is that they omit certain essential elements. Women in their forties often seem to suffer from poor nutrition, especially those who have indulged in crash diets.They then need more protein and extra vitamins to counteract their deficiencies.

Other rather suspicious weight control methods have been or still are popular. One dubious way to lose weight "dramatically" is by means of injecting placental extract daily, and at the same time maintaining a 500-calorie daily diet. The value of the placental extract has not been verified, and it is clear enough that on a 500-calorie diet weight would be lost in any event.

In some cases (fortunately few!), dental surgeons have been willing to sew the mouths of their patients closed, to prevent them from eating. No comment is needed on such extreme techniques.

Massage for weight reduction—as well as for exercise—is ineffective. There is no true evidence that it "breaks up fat so it will dissolve," and the idea of massage in particular spots to reduce them is even more senseless.

Advertisements appear from time to time for creams, massage garments, liquids in which to soak garments, and an assortment of other equally fraudulent impositions on the will-to-believe.

The Best Diets

The best diets are simple and unspectacular and produce permanent weight loss. Continual weight jumps or losses are wearing on the system and it is better to concentrate on *maintaining* weight if you feel you will only regain the weight you've taken off. Here are six tips for a sound diet.

1. To maintain weight the menopausal woman needs about fourteen calories per pound.
2. Any reducing diet for the menopausal woman should contain adequate calcium and vitamin D. And the calcium should be obtained from a low-fat source: skimmed milk or pot cheese.
3. Protein is important: again, low-fat sources, such as fish, lean meat, and soy beans, are best.
4. Leafy green vegetables, salads, fruit, fruit juice—one of this group twice daily.
5. Whole-grain breads or cereals, or legumes such as lima beans, kidney beans, or lentils provide valuable B vitamins.
6. Salt intake should be limited somewhat in menopausal women.

EXERCISE

Life for prehistoric people was rigorous and active, and human bodies evolved to meet the demands of an often precarious existence as hunter or hunted. We are designed to *need* exercise. Without it our muscles wither away. Our bones become soft and more brittle, even our spirits sink and our level of nervous tension increases. In earlier cultures, as life became less strenuous, more formal ways of exercising developed. In early societies, dance expressed the body's need to move and to be expressive. For example, in Polynesia the dance became a language to express emotions and tell stories, as well as to serve a religious function. Early cultures also created systems of exercise to prepare for tribal defense or individual combat, or to demonstrate athletic skills. Our modern systems of exercises grew out of a Swedish method of gymnastics first published in 1860, designed to keep the army and farm workers physically fit. The Swedish model became the basis of calisthenics programs throughout northern Europe and the United States. But, although we pay lip service to the need for exercise for our school children, we are still a fairly sedentary nation. Lately, there has been a growing interest in sports and physical development for young women, and this trend is all to the good. But what about women of menopausal age?

WHY EXERCISE NOW?

Exercise is of vital importance to women as a means of delaying or even preventing some aspects of aging of the body. It improves the circulation of the blood and the tone of all the muscles, including the diaphragm and the heart. In fact, cardiologists have come to view exercise as a necessity in preventing aging of the heart muscle. Exercise also benefits the gastrointestinal tract and aids bowel function. A well-exercised person has better posture and a more youthful, more vigorous appearance. Relaxation, better sleep, and a general sense of well-being are the rewards of exercise.

By lowering body weight and by burning up sugar, exercise aids in lowering cholesterol. If you are still unconvinced of the need to exercise, read the following grim portrait.

An underexercised older woman ages more rapidly and more extensively. Her bones lose calcium more quickly and become fragile, and her torso tends to bend forward as the spine softens and curves. Her stature decreases. Her cartilage hardens faster, resulting in stiffer joints, and her flabby muscles cannot maintain good posture. This allows the normal thickening of her torso to be greatly exaggerated and her stomach protrudes. There is no reason why this should happen, for it is the inevitable consequence not of age but of inactivity.

Obviously, there are immense benefits to exercise, but how should you get started, especially if you've been fairly sedentary up until now? Should you choose a formal program or follow your own? You know yourself best. If you find it difficult to plan a schedule and adhere to it, if you are stimulated by a group atmosphere and find supervision helpful, by all means join a group you like. If you can make a plan and can discipline yourself, there is no reason why you can't select the exercises you prefer and do them on your own, informally.

CHOOSING YOUR OWN WAY TO EXERCISE

There are many ways to exercise, ranging from dancing to formal calisthenics to informal hiking. The best daily all-around exercise (and the easiest to do) is brisk walking (a mile in fifteen minutes) for several miles, if possible. Swimming, bicycling, horseback riding, skating, golf (without a cart), skiing, gardening, and tennis are all good and enjoyable. Hiking with a group such as the Sierra Club is great exercise and offers additional advantages of a social and spiritual sort.

Be wary of belly dancing, which may cause back sprains, and of jogging, if you're not in good shape or if you'd be running on hard city streets. If you have disc problems or osteoarthritis of the spine (common in older women) jogging will cause further damage.

Before taking up any of the more formal or strenuous exercise programs, the menopausal or older woman should have a physical examination or stress test, especially if she has any cardiac or hypertensive history.

A stress test can be done in many ways. The simplest is to have you walk on a treadmill to the limits of your endurance while a constant check is made of your pulse rate and blood pressure. If these approach a dangerously high level or if an attached electrocardiogram shows the beginning of abnormal wave changes, you have reached your maximal level of stress and should exercise below that. The physician can evaluate those capable of doing mild, moderate, or strenuous exercise by the length of time it takes to produce stress.

All exercises should be started slowly and gradually increased in length and strenuousness. They should always be stopped if vertigo or chest pain develops.

GOOD WAYS TO EXERCISE IN COMPANY

Modern dance, ballet, and yoga taught by well-trained instructors are fine exercises and fun to do. Yoga can also, once taught, be done alone. It helps breathing and relaxation and promotes mobility as well as the stretching and strengthening of muscles.

Gymnasium and health club programs, which offer proper medical supervision for individual needs, can provide a wide range of calisthenics, dance, and sports. The YWCA is especially noteworthy for its good medical provisions and skilled instructors.

EXERCISING ON YOUR OWN

If you prefer to do it yourself, there are any number of exercises you can perform at home. The kinds of exercise you need are those that stimulate breathing and heart action, muscle strength and overall flexibility. One good system is the Canadian Air Force exercises. You should plan to eliminate push-ups because these put too much pressure on the spine. Isometric exercises tone muscles but do not provide stimulation of lungs and heart. Therefore, they should only be part of an overall program.

The following list of exercises is designed to keep you fit in a number of ways. These are not strenuous and are suitable for women who haven't been especially active. Depending on your condition, the extent to which you have exercised previously, and individual medical recommendations, you may choose from the following exercises which emphasize strength and stretching. Variety is to be recommended. Plan to start by spending ten minutes a day, gradually working up to forty-five minutes.

1. Running in place, or around a room. Note that running at home, with its saving of time, its lack of special clothing requirements, and its all-weather availability, is just as beneficial as running (or jogging) outdoors.

2. Lie on your back, knees slightly bent. Catch feet securely under a bed, couch, cabinet, or heavy chair. Clasp hands behind head. Rise to sitting position, return to reclining position.

3. Lie flat, arms at sides. Raise left leg straight up. Lower. Repeat with right leg.

4. Repeat exercise 3, but when each leg is raised, swing it slowly to one side and back up, then lower it to floor.

5. Lie flat. Raise left knee with clasped hands. Raise head until you can "kiss" your knee. Repeat with right knee.

6. Stand, place your hands flat against each other as if in prayer. Push them against each other as hard as you can.

7. Lie down, knees flexed, soles on floor. Extend left leg as far as you can, pointing toe. Return to flexed position and let go limply. Repeat with right leg.

158 | THE MENOPAUSE BOOK

8. Lie on left side, knees flexed. Extend right leg as far as you can, return to flexed position, let go limply. Repeat lying on right side, stretching left leg.

9. Assume position on all fours, resting palms and knees on floor. Raise back the way a cat stretches, then lower abdomen in a reverse movement. Repeat several times.

10. Sit on floor cross-legged. Reach as *high* as you can with right hand, then left hand. Repeat starting with left hand.

11. Sit cross-legged on floor. Reach out *forward* as far as you can with left hand. Repeat with right hand.

12. Stand on tiptoes, rock back and forth from heels to toes.

13. Stand straight. Keeping knees straight, bend to touch floor with fingertips.

14. Stand straight, reach for ceiling with both hands.

TEN AIDS FOR SUCCESSFUL EXERCISE

1. Expect to *enjoy* it. (Don't regard it grimly as a duty!) It's vital not only for health, but also for a renewal from the routines of living. You'll return to them feeling better!

2. You *do* have time. You can't afford *not* to. And it takes very little.

3. Start *now* (read the rest of this list when you've finished). Put it down for *almost* every day, on your calendar. A new habit needs conscious effort, especially at first. And don't let exceptions occur unless, of course, you're feeling ill.

4. Start slowly, increase gradually. The Sierra Club hikes are carefully classified as "easy," "moderate," and "strenuous." The Canadian Air Force program is admirable for its assignment of exercises related to age and its stress on gradual increments.

5. Compare what you do each day with what *you* did yesterday. (Don't compare yourself with your most athletic friend or a professional athlete!)

6. Don't be a hero. Listen to your body. Warning signs are dizziness, shortness of breath, muscle tension, trembling, fatigue, pain. When one of these signals appears, stop! Be especially careful in very hot and cold windy weather. (Start slowly when it's cold.)

7. Watch for opportunities to exercise. Whenever you can, walk instead of riding. You might get off the bus or subway a little before your destination, climb a flight of stairs instead of using the elevator. You'll discover other ways, too.

8. Find ways to make exercise more amusing. Remember that for some, a competitive sport or game is more interesting than a calisthenic routine. Keep track of your growing accomplishments. Can you swim more and more laps, raise your leg higher and straighter, bend more flexibly as the weeks go by? This "knowledge of results" adds definite interest to exercising.

9. If you exercise alone, do it to music for fun or with a radio news program to keep you company.

10. Remember: Massage is good only for developing the muscles of the masseuse. It's fine for relaxation and pleasure, but only your own efforts will strengthen you. That's why machines at health clubs aren't really helpful.

To sum up, a physically fit woman of fifty should plan to spend about fifteen minutes a day exercising in addition to creating a lifestyle that includes plenty of walking. Exercise classes, modern dance, folk dance, yoga, and gymnastics are all good forms of exercise—and, one last thought, so is making love. For this, there is no age limit.

HYPERTENSION

Hypertension, or high blood pressure, occurs when the arterioles become abnormally narrow, forcing the heart to work harder in order to pump blood. If there is *constant* high pressure, the heart and arterial system is subjected to greatly increased wear and tear from the heavier pounding with each pulse beat. Hypertension must be followed by a physician and if not controlled by diet, exercise, or relaxation, should be treated with appropriate drugs. It can lead to strokes, heart attacks, and kidney failure.

About 20 percent of the adult population over forty has this condition, although it is not age related; it may occur in much younger people and go undiagnosed for years. Yet, properly treated, it is a disease that most often is successfully controlled. Often, hypertension makes its first appearance at menopause, a time of stress and physical change.

If your physical examination reveals the presence of high blood pressure, there are several things your doctor may suggest. He or she may ask you to restrict your salt intake, something already suggested in this chapter as a general measure. A low-salt diet will help eliminate excess fluids from the body, thereby relieving pressure. If you are overweight, your doctor may suggest a reducing diet. You may also be given medication which will lower your blood pressure.

If emotional stress or tension appears to be a factor in your case, there are various ways of reducing or controlling it.

RELAXATION

General relaxation can often be achieved with a conscious effort to think (or meditate) calmly. Women who are feeling tense and anxious should spend ten minutes twice a day, sitting or lying down, by themselves, with the door shut. During this period they should shut out thoughts of the world around them, chores, household routines, job duties, bills, etc. They should concentrate on the "here and now," not the past or the future. This requires practice. It may help to select a single image on which to concentrate in each of these ten-minute periods: a flower, a pleasant perfume, your hands—even a spot on the wall. Try to be aware of the way you feel when you do achieve relaxation—and contrast that feeling with those of tension and anxiety. The ability to relax consciously is one we learn slowly, so don't be disappointed if you can't do it at once.

Transcendental meditation is a formal relaxation program that appeals to the religiously or mystically inclined person. The object or thought on which one concentrates is called a *mantra*, and formal training in relaxation is carried out at TM centers. Many people have enjoyed learning relaxation techniques in this way; however, there is evidence that similar results are obtained simply by following an informal approach on your own.

Another method of relaxing tension—and, indirectly, blood pressure—is the use of biofeedback apparatus designed for that purpose. The subject sees her blood pressure reading on a dial. She is instructed to remember an unusually peaceful, enjoyable moment, and then watches for a drop in the blood pressure reading following this. She may also detect less muscular tension and less anxiety. In this way, with repeated trials, she may train herself to control a bodily response (blood pressure) not ordinarily subject to voluntary alteration. Again, there is evidence that similar beneficial changes can be induced by thinking peaceful thoughts without using any apparatus. Relaxation should be something you practice for a short time every day.

Some Specific Exercises

As part of a medical approach to lowering blood pressure and relieving stress and anxiety, the following physical exercises are designed to be used almost anywhere—at home or in the office—and you need ten minutes at most to do them.

1. Sit on the edge of a chair, couch, or bed. Raise your right hand forward, hold at shoulder height until it aches. Let it drop to your lap. Notice both the previously tense, and later relaxed sensation in your muscles, a feeling of physical and mental ease. Repeat with your left hand.

2. Sit on the edge of a chair, couch, or bed. Lift your right leg, holding it out until it aches. Let your heel drop to the floor. Observe the previously tense, later relaxed sensations, which then begin to spread to other parts of your body. Repeat with your left leg.

3. Contact your face and neck muscles until they ache. Let go. Study your sensations as the relieved feeling spreads.

4. Sit as above, and contract your buttocks muscles. Let go.

5. Sit as above, and contract the muscles above your knees. Let go.

6. Breathe in deeply. Exhale slowly.

As you do these relaxation exercises you'll become more and more familiar with the tensed sensations before, and the relaxed sensations after, each exercise in each part of the body. Such relaxation tends to spread, and brings with it mental relaxation as well. Muscles are often far more tense than they need be to walk, drive, or talk to people. You can learn to release that tension in everyday life, and thus extend the benefits of the exercises to all your activities.

Other Tension Treatments

An additional way to deal with anxiety (if it is attached to some realistic cause for concern) is the "action cure" for worry. If you have the habit of worrying about your work (home, bills, children), focus on what you can *do* about the problem, and *do it*.

Autosuggestion is still another tension treatment. Actually *say* to yourself: "I will be calm. I will be at peace with myself. Life simply is not worthwile if I worry so much." This simple method is often remarkably potent.

COSMETIC SURGERY

As the years pass and the signs of age appear, most women feel an understandable concern. No doubt this concern is exaggerated by our society's worship of youthful good looks. There are normal changes in appearance due to age—changes in muscle firmness, shape of the breasts, distribution of body weight, fat distribution. Looking in the mirror we see blemishes, wrinkles, pouches. Women at menopause often wonder whether or not cosmetic surgery could delay such changes or restore youthful characteristics. Unlike any other kind of surgery, there is no health reason to have your face lifted or your breasts reshaped. How do women go about making the decision to have a purely cosmetic operation?

YOUR BODY IMAGE AND YOUR PERSONALITY

An important part of your personality depends on how you *feel* about your body. An attractive woman can identify her entire being with her physical appearance. The woman who is convinced that her appearance has serious flaws may identify with these and feel insecure. Certainly, if you feel discontented with some aspect of your physique or physiognomy, you should *consider* what cosmetic surgery might accomplish. The rewards can be great, but the decision is weighty. I have patients whose lives have been brightened by it. One woman who is not really pretty had a simple cosmetic operation done for a receding chin. Because she feels so pleased with the effect, she radiates joy and the sense of well-being of a great beauty. I also have patients who wish they had never heard of it.

WHO MAKES THE DECISION?

The decision should be made by three people.

You, of course, are the main person concerned, and almost always you would be the one to raise the question. It is possible, too, that your own physician, noting a need, would suggest it. In any event he or she is the one most familiar with you as a person and with your health, and should play a part. The third person is the specialist, the cosmetic surgeon.

Your own doctor may be able to recommend an able surgeon in whom he has complete confidence. A friend whose judgment you trust might have a name to suggest. Your local County Medical Society, or a fully staffed voluntary hospital, will offer you several names from which to make your own selection. Check to see if the surgeon you intend to use has been certified as competent by a reliable organization: Two that certify proficiency in cosmetic surgery are the American Board of Plastic Surgery and the American Society of Plastic and Reconstructive Surgeons. In asking for a recommendation and seeking assurance, it is wise to specify the type of surgery required: facial, head, hands, etc. Each area requires specialized training.

WHEN IS IT BENEFICIAL?

Women whose occupations require a youthful appearance—models, for instance, and actresses—have the most obvious reasons to turn to cosmetic surgery. The added years made possible in such occupations and others are of major importance.

Some women have "fantasy defects," something about the nose, ears, or eyes which they believe is disfiguring but which does not appear so to others, the kind of thing no reasonable persons would worry about. Unfortunately, the neurotic woman who should not have cosmetic surgery may pursue her goal with such determination that eventually some surgeon will give in and operate against his better judgment. No surgeon should operate *solely on demand*; he should do so only when the request seems soundly based.

WHAT IT CAN AND CANNOT DO

The outstanding benefit of cosmetic surgery is a physical appearance so much improved that a woman can identify with it to great advantage, feel more comfortable about herself and more assured with others.

But no surgical or other medical process can halt the aging process. This may seem too obvious to mention, but so strong is the eternal quest for youth that some women are willfully unrealistic. Unreasonable expectations may create a major problem. The first type of unrealistic hope is that the procedure will make a plain face beautiful. A woman in her middle fifties recently asked an opinion about the removal of rather prominent fat deposits near her eyes. The project seemed reasonable, so she was referred to a cosmetic surgeon who discussed the procedure with her. However, midway through the conversation the woman produced a photograph of a woman half her age and considerably prettier, with enormous, beautiful eyes. Pointing to the picture she announced that that was her objective! The surgeon courteously declined to operate and explained that because her expectations were far too unreal, she was bound to be bitterly disappointed.

A second type of unrealistic expectation is the hope that the repair will last indefinitely. Except in the case of certain bone operations, this is utterly impossible.

A third type of unrealistic expectation is the belief that the operation will change the course of one's life. The distinction between the dream and the reality is expressed in such terms as these: "If I have my nose changed, my whole life will improve." "I feel so inferior. If the double chin is removed, I'll be a new person!" I'll never get older!" "I'll be fascinating looking. My conversation will improve. Men will admire me. Everyone will take notice!"

With skill and good fortune an operable *defect* will be remedied or lessened, but one's personality will remain the same and friends and relatives may not notice a definite change. There was a case in which one man, who was away while his wife had a face-lift, was completely unaware of any change until she mentioned it. In another case a woman's friends thought she looked better and well rested but didn't know why.

WHO SHOULD NOT HAVE COSMETIC SURGERY

All surgery and procedures requiring anesthesia have risks, even if they are usually minimal. In cosmetic surgery, local anesthesia is usually used, but even this risk is prohibitive for a woman with uncontrolled diabetes, uncontrolled high blood pressure, any severely debilitating disease, or a tendency to bleed.

Asiatic and black women do not develop wrinkles or sagging musculature of the face the way white women do. Therefore, these groups almost never need facial surgery. Because black skin has a marked tendency to develop keloids (large, thick scars), black women have an additional reason to avoid such cosmetic surgery.

IMPROVING SKIN THROUGH SURGERY

There are several procedures facial surgeons use to remove superficial lines and wrinkles and improve the texture of the skin. Each method entails definite risks, causes pain, and often costs quite a lot of money. Before undergoing any of these procedures, you should discuss it thoroughly with your doctor.

Face Peels

To smooth away superficial facial wrinkles and lines, "chemical surgery" is a possible—but, some doctors feel, an unjustifiably risky—procedure. (Skin below the face is entirely unsuitable for this method.) A caustic agent called phenol (carbolic acid) is swabbed or brushed on and literally burns the top facial skin layers. Since the hours immediately following are painful, sedatives are customary. Successful treatment brings recovery after about two weeks, with the expectation that the improved skin will last several years.

There are strict limitations and precautions connected with face peeling: blue-eyed blond women are the best prospects, whereas dark-complexioned subjects are regarded as definite risks. Black women should never have it as it may cause bad scars and areas of depigmentation. A preliminary examination is an absolute necessity, to rule out women with diabetes or liver, heart, or kidney disease, as well as any with a marked tendency toward scarring. Possible dangers which the patient faces are kidney damage and/or failure due to the phenol, coarsened skin, white blotches, scars, and serious effects on the nervous system, respiratory tract, and muscles. A few women have died from the effects of phenol.

In my opinion, the face peel is almost always inadvisable. The relatively slight facial conditions to be corrected, the limitation on who is a good risk, as well as the pain and discomfort involved—all deserve the most careful evaluation. Skin color is not divided absolutely into blond and brunette, nor are diseases either fully present or completely absent in all cases. There are many degrees of risk. Face peeling requires great skill, and the most careful precautions are essential. Burning one's face is not a trivial decision and the results are sometimes unattractive. Some faces so treated look taut and strange and oddly shiny, as if they had been severely burned—as was indeed the case.

Dermaplaning

The dermatone is a surgical tool, similar in its action to the carpenter's plane. It removes an extremely thin slice of facial skin in order to permit new and presumably more attractive skin to replace it. (Surgeons use this to obtain a patch of skin for performing a skin graft.) The procedure is painful even with sedation and postoperative medication. Most patients are horrified by their appearance for two weeks or so after surgery. Good results are obtained by the most highly skilled surgeons. Once you have undergone this procedure, you must absolutely stay out of the sun or run the risk of developing unattractive pigmentation!

Cryosurgery

Freezing is used to destroy superficial facial skin and with it a variety of defects such as birthmarks and warts. Liquid nitrogen at extremely low temperature is used for this purpose. Freezing, too, is painful, must be performed by a skilled surgeon, and requires a decision to stay out of the sun.

Dermabrasion

An alternative method for removing or ameliorating defects such as wrinkles and scars is by means of an electrically powered, rapidly rotating wire brush. As in the other methods described, the purpose is to destroy top skin layers and permit new growth. Sandpaper applied by hand has a similar effect. Local or a general anesthesia is employed, and recovery time is about two weeks. Many of my patients have achieved a smoother, younger skin with dermabrasion. They all say that on the next day they wondered why they had ever done it, but after a few weeks were very much pleased with the result. Of course, the method cannot completely erase deep scars or pits of acne, since it can only be superficial.

Altering Facial Features

Cosmetic surgery has been applied to alter thick lips or change the contour of a nose (sometimes merely because it had an unwanted ethnic association), install dimples, raise, alter, or create eyebrows, and increase the number of eyelashes. Unless there is an unusually compelling reason to undego the risks of surgery, it is felt that such procedures are unjustifiable, approaching the trivial or even frivolous and grotesque.

Face-Lifts

Our faces all age differently—and we all feel differently about those changes that we experience. Depending on the degree of aging, some women want to reverse these effects by having a face-lift—to tighten or eradicate a drooping chin, jowls, eyelid wrinkles, bags beneath the eyes, and unsightly fatty accumulations. Sometimes corrections of eye defects can be a separate procedure from the face-lift, or can be combined with it in a longer operation. (Lifting of the neck is typically an accompaniment.)

A skilled surgeon makes a great effort to operate in such a way that scars are minimized and obscured by the hairline and placed in unobtrusive locations near the ears and by the neck. Loose folds of skin are excised; muscles are adjusted for increased tone. The practice of inserting silicone in solid form to remodel the face is inadvisable, for the silicone may shift around. A face-lift is performed in a well-equipped hospital operating room, and you should expect a stay of about four days. Before the operation, the patient is given a sedative, and during the procedure local anesthesia is used because the surgeon needs the patient's cooperation to get the best results. Patients are given medication for postoperative pain and may need it for some time. (Remember that it takes time to feel pain, time to inform a nurse or the doctor even in a hospital, and time to obtain pain-relieving medication. When you are back home and telephone the doctor, he or she is not always sitting at the telephone.)

It takes at least a week before you can resume your usual activities, and for a while you'll need cosmetics to cover the redness.

The benefits of a face-life last about five or six years, but signs of aging gradually begin to return before that approximate date.

Cosmetic Surgery for the Breast

At menopause the breasts normally shrink or become pendulous. Surgery has been developed that will reshape breast contours. For example, to increase the size of the breast and adjust its shape, the surgeon makes an incision beneath the breast so that the scar will be covered and then implants a silicone rubber envelope filled with silicone gel into a pocket incised for that purpose. Feelings of tension and pain commonly follow the operation and may last several weeks. To reduce the size of a larger or pendulous breast, the surgeon removes suitable amounts of skin, fat, and other tissue. Hospitalization for four days is usual after these procedures, and general anesthesia is preferred. Postoperative activity must be restricted. Such procedures are warranted only in the most extreme cases. Silicone implants may mask the symptoms of early breast cancer and delay detection.

Cosmetic Body Surgery

Women have sought surgical correction for an assortment of conditions: excess fat on thighs, buttocks, arms, and waist; extra folds of skin and the pendulous "apron of fat" across the abdomen. Risks exist from possible infection, from hemorrhage, and from embolisms caused by fat entering the bloodstream. Before attempting an operation the physician would recommend a program of exercise and weight loss.

Surgical correction of unsightly veins and wrinkles on the hands is a serious procedure. These would have to be unusually disfiguring before such an operation could be recommended.

ALL SURGERY IS SERIOUS

Women should always regard cosmetic surgery as a major enterprise and expect their doctors to give it the most cautious and conservative consideration before recommending it. There comes to mind the case of a woman who was strongly advised by a careful and responsible surgeon *not* to have surgical correction for excess fat in her arms, thighs, and abdomen. She finally found a surgeon who would perform the operation and lost about 100 pounds on the operating table. After recovery from surgery, she returned to her old eating habits and in five months regained the 100 pounds and more. She is someone who might have benefited from a psychiatric consultation. She needed to restructure her abnormal eating habits; her expensive, painful, disfiguring experience was all for nothing.

Cosmetic surgery is not to be undertaken lightly. It is not completely safe, not always effective, and not always painless. Wishful thinking by the patient and a disarmingly cheerful manner on the part of the surgeon can be a most unfortunate combination.

HAIR

Thinning of hair is a universal problem and occurs to some degree in all women at the time of menopause. It is better not to use a hairbrush because it is easy to pull out hair follicles. A gentle combing is sufficient. As you age, your hair loses oil so it should be washed less frequently—once a week is enough. Cream rinses and other products that untangle hair are good because the hair can then be combed out without much pulling. Detergent shampoos should be avoided because they are drying to the scalp. Castile soap is still one of the best products for washing hair.

If hair seems excessively thin, one's thyroid activity should be checked. At the time of menopause, many women experience a decrease in thyroid production, and if this is the problem thyroid tablets taken daily will usually help; after a few months the hair will begin to grow and thicken.

Women should be wary of heat treatments or light treatments for the hair; they usually prove worthless. Both estrogen and cortisone have been applied to the scalp in an effort to increase growth of hair in menopausal women, but they don't work. Oral estrogen has been used for this purpose but to take estrogen solely for thinning hair is questionable.

SKIN CARE

As we get older the skin has less oil, and we would be wise to use a moisturizer. Soap and water are still essential. Wash your face at least once a day with a moderately rough washcloth and a good non-alkaline soap to get rid of superficial scaling and extra cells and then apply a moisturizer. An inexpensive one such as Albolene is just as good as the wildly expensive creams sold in fancy packages. All makeup should be completely washed off with soap and water before applying the moisturizer.

Good nutrition is most important to maintaining good skin. Vitamin supplements help. Some women have had good results with 10,000 units of Vitamin A, 500 milligrams of Vitamin C, and one Vitamin B-complex capsule. Larger doses taken daily can create toxic effects.

Unfortunately, there are many more don'ts than dos in regard to care for skin at the time of menopause. Vigorous massages and costly facial treatments at beauty parlors can be actually harmful to skin, particularly if a woman's skin has always been sensitive. Vacuums can actually rupture superficial blood vessels, leaving a permanent blotchy effect.

In addition, many dermatologists are beginning to question the positive effects of facial exercises. Often, instead of strengthening the facial muscles they create wrinkles—especially around the mouth and eyes.

Every dermatologist agrees that besides the normal toll of years the sun is the greatest enemy of smooth skin. The best way to keep skin looking young is to avoid the sun. Wear a broad-brimmed hat and dark glasses for protection in strong sunlight.

It may also be necessary to cover up at the beach because sunlight causes problems for all skin, not just facial skin. Liver spots are direct products of the sun and are somewhat difficult to remove. There are two ways to remove them. One method, an acid treatment, must be applied very carefully since the acid may leave a scar or a depigmented area. The other method, an application of Quinone derivatives, can be irritating and also cause a complete depigmentation, so a dark spot is only replaced with a white spot. Keratoses (horny patches of skin) are not as serious and can be removed by a dermatologist quite successfully with a minimum of effort. The best advice is to stay out of strong sun as much as possible.

Aging skin is also affected by extreme exposure to heat and cold. As you grow older, saunas and facial saunas can be very bad for your skin because extreme cold and extreme heat may be excessively drying.

THE OVERALL GOAL

The real purpose toward which all the advice in this chapter is aimed is not to deprive you of pleasure through the rigors of diet and exercise, the warnings against smoking and drinking and cautions against the sun. The goal is to help you look and feel good. Exercise in itself is pleasurable. Having a strong body is pleasurable and possible. Cutting down on smoking and drinking increases a sense of physical well-being and improves your chances to be and remain healthy. Use the information in this chapter to increase your sense of well-being and your confidence in your body, in its strength and attractiveness. Women can be beautiful at any age, but as they grow older that beauty resides in vitality and intelligence as much as in skin texture or regular features. Women today, more than ever before, have the knowledge and opportunity to develop both kinds of beauty.

10

WOMEN TALK ABOUT MENOPAUSE

The women we interviewed for this chapter are a varied group in personality, education, and life-styles. There are widows, married women, women with and without children, a single woman, and a woman long separated from her husband. Some work, some do not. Some have had great difficulty with menopause and some have not.

We asked them specific questions about menopause and more general questions about their lives in order to help you understand how menopause affected them in what they were doing and what prejudices they brought to the experience.

All these women were raised by sexually repressed and repressive mothers, themselves victims of Victorian upbringings. Periods were "the curse," and one spoke about them as little as possible. Menopause seems to have been even less of a topic for discussion; little or no information on any aspect of sexuality was passed along from one generation to the next.

In retrospect, it seems amazing that mothers could have so little to tell their daughters. They were ready to insist that the most important thing a woman could be was a wife and mother, and yet, when it came to practical information about being a woman, nothing was said or shared. No mother told her daughter how to have sex, how to give birth, or how to prepare for the time of life when she would have menopause.

For the most part, the women we interviewed came to menopause knowing little about their bodies in general and the psychobiological changes in particular that women experience. Their doctors did little to educate them.

Some of these women have made great changes in their lives. One went to graduate school at fifty; several others returned to work—or began working for the first time—when their children had grown. The biggest changes that they have faced, though, seem to be changes associated with aging rather than any emotional difficulties related to the loss of childbearing ability.

As you read this chapter, some of the varied feelings and problems discussed in these interviews will sound familiar. You may identify with one or more of these women or you may disagree with the way they draw conclusions. But we hope that as you read these women's own words for their own experiences, you will feel that your problems are shared by others and that whatever your particular experience of menopause, there is someone else out there who knows what you mean.

INTERVIEW 1

"My mother was an ardent feminist all her life, but I felt that family life was pretty interesting."

The subject of the first interview followed a pattern typical of the many women who married around the time of World War II. After getting her college degree, she married and raised a family. Like many suburban women she spent time doing volunteer work—but with a special intensity and energy. Later, she was able to use the skills she had developed in community work to develop an interesting career. At age fifty, she took a professional degree and now holds a rewarding and demanding job. Menopause was a nuisance for this energetic woman because of the discomfort caused by hot flashes, but it was not a change that has posed any emotional problems.

"I can't think of anything more intellectually stimulating and exciting than watching a kid grow up and being involved in the process. I just loved being the mother of small kids. I never felt put upon by society or that I wasn't really working; in fact, I was as busy as hell.

"As my kids went off to school I got more and more involved in local political problems, and I worked very hard on many local elections and was involved in various school study groups. I felt very deeply about improving and supporting public schools, and about getting other people to support them. These activities and others, including the Girl Scouts, took a huge amount of my time. After my school phase, in 1960, I got reinvolved with an organization for exchange students. For about eight years, I organized a student exchange program in the area of Ohio in which we lived. I would go into communities, seek out the community leaders, and get them interested enough to raise money for local programs. I organized about sixteen small-town programs and I found the work fascinating. I could work from home and do as much work as I wanted. I used to work, on the average, sixty hours a week. I had to touch base with the state organization every so often and report on my progress and they were happy as clams. I found the different phases of this work absorbing: going into the communities; working with the volunteers; organizing different setups so that they would survive for at least a year or two; and publicizing them. Although I wasn't paid for my time, I did acquire a lot of skills. It was very responsible work, and in many ways I find it was the most satisfying work experience I have had. I am not condescending toward volunteers, because being one can be very rewarding.

"After the children grew up we moved to Chicago, and I began to look around for other things to do. By a fluke I fell into a job working for the city government as executive director of a small office that worked with representatives of foreign governments, who were based in the city. I used a lot of the skills that I had learned as a volunteer. A very dominating, brilliant, person whom I found difficult to work with was in charge of the whole operation. After a year, I left. This was in 1970. There was a serious recession at the time and funding for all international programs was cut back; their staffs were cut in half and there was no more hiring. I knew I had a lot of skills, but the only thing I had had any experience in was the work I'd been doing. After trying for about a year to find a job, I decided that what I needed was a skill that could be independent of advancing age. By the time I entered graduate school I was fifty.

"It was the fall of 1971 and my youngest child had graduated from college that past spring. I enrolled in a full-time graduate program in city planning. I have a very helpful husband in all ways. He paid the way and was understanding of the time it took. It took me a long time to get my degree, and we really gave up almost all of our social life.

"I was the oldest person in my class and in the school. Most of the students were the age of my children, but I had always enjoyed my children and their friends.

"My classmates treated me extremely decently and were not a bit patronizing. They sensitized me and raised by consciousness on the issues of women to such an extent that I now feel mildly insulted if a man holds a door open for me.

"The younger people seemed to know how to take exams better than I did, but I don't think that has anything to do with age. I suppose they were a little more used to studying, but I had been working all that time in other ways.

"After the end of the first year, I noticed a plea from the student association for student members of various faculty committees—we were sort of the last activist class. I thought, 'What the hell, I'll apply.' I was one of five student members of a faculty committee for the next two years. The professors were younger than I was. At the beginning I was definitely part of the older generation; but by the second year, I began to notice I was always voting for the students against the faculty. It was very interesting; out of conviction I was totally on their side. At the end of three years, I felt it was "us against them." Generation had nothing to do with it.

"It gave me a much better understanding of my childrens' generation and their attitudes.

"Since leaving graduate school, I've been working for two years for a community project in neighborhood revitalization. One of our projects is a complaint center for people to call in with all sorts of problems—landlord/tenant problems, problems with government agencies, etc. We try to help no matter what the problem is. I've just gotten a promotion, which will involve organizing on a much larger scale.

"During my graduate training, I realized that my periods were changing. In my late thirties I had started having abnormally long periods—often with blood clots. At times it seemed as if I was practically hemorrhaging, which was particularly distressing. Finally, my doctor told me that I needed a D and C, which would stop the excessive bleeding. Over a period of seven years, I had to have three D and Cs.

Later, I began to notice that I would occasionally skip a period. I continued to skip one or two periods and would then have a fairly normal period and then skip again.

"But I really didn't have many concerns about menopause until I was about forty-seven, when I began to have hot flashes, which were and still are the only part of the whole process that I have found physically distressing. Distressing may be too strong a word. But they are really annoying. I went to a gynecologist regularly and he started me out on very, very minimal doses of oral estrogen. My doctor felt that, while this kind of medication was often helpful, people took too much of it and for too long. He liked to start with a minimal dose and work up. I took estrogen for quite a while, increasing the doses to two and even three times as much but I never reached the high level some people take. Estrogen certainly did help; I didn't experience any side effects, and I stopped having hot flashes. At one point either that doctor or another doctor suggested I stop taking it entirely, which I did. I also thought it was time. Then I started having hot flashes again. It went back and forth like this for a while.

"When I read all that stuff about estrogens, I just stopped. I thought what little discomfort I was having wasn't worth the risk. At that point I was waking up three or four times a night with hot flashes. That was nothing compared to what it had been before, which was every half hour. Before I had experienced flashes, I had always felt they were psychological. But once, I went to have an electroencephalograph, and during the procedure I had a hot flash and didn't mention it. The doctor said, 'Oh, for God sakes, you're getting hot flashes, aren't you?' And I said, 'Yes, but it never occurred to me that you would be able to detect it.' He said, 'Of course I can.' I think this is because your skin really gets very hot and the electrodes on your skin register the heat. It changed the brain wave pattern, too; it looked like an earthquake.

"When I was going to school the hot flashes were very disturbing. In the middle of class I'd find myself rolling up my sleeves. It may be that I feel more uncomfortable than most because I sweat so minimally.

"I don't know whether my mother had hot flashes or not. She was a very reticent and puritanical lady and found it difficult to discuss anything sexual. Also she is a good deal older than I; she was probably well into menopause by the time I started menstruating. By the time

I hit my own menopause, mother was very old, sort of off in another world.

"I think a great deal—too much—is made about menopause. I haven't found it particularly distressing except for the hot flashes.

"You do miss your kids when they grow up and leave the nest. I used to go to the mailbox every day to see if there was a letter. But after a short time you get used to them being away and you get busy doing something else. Days go by without your even thinking about them. Then the kids come back and visit and you have a lovely time. When they go off, you miss them again for about a week, and then you become reinvolved with something else. It works the other way too. If they come and stay a little too long, really, you can't wait to get rid of them. I adore them, but we are all adults and work in different modes, and we are just not set up to live together. I suppose if we had to, we would adjust to it.

"Most other aspects of menopause have not been particularly unpleasant for me. Your body changes as you grow older. I remember when I got my first gray hair or two—but after a while I got so I liked gray hair. Again, it is a problem of seeing yourself. I think it is very hard to see yourself, even in the mirror, because you are still in that business of being inside your own body, and it changes so slowly. I occasionally see myself in a photograph that somebody has taken and I think, 'Oh my God, what jowls.' I don't think of myself as jowly, and it takes a little while to get used to the idea that I have jowls.

"I have always felt that my husband found me terribly attractive at each stage of my life, and I think a lot of my jolly attitude stems from having such a nice husband. I think we have an exceptionally nice relationship. I am very pro-marriage. It is a very fulfilling relationship, and it is nice to grow old together.

"I do feel very strongly, although I don't have any actual proof of it, that there is discrimination against people because of their age. I felt this when I first went job hunting at age fifty-three. The employer feels that he can't offer an older woman a bottom-rung job, because she is experienced. It takes a really gutsy guy like the one who hired me to see that he could use me effectively. When various agencies posted openings, I went and applied but I wasn't offered any of those jobs. One of the employers almost said that he wouldn't dream of hiring a woman of my age. It was made very clear to me what the problem was. I said, 'Well, why not?' 'Well,' he said, 'we don't hire anyone unless that person will be staying with us long enough to become executive director.' I told him I was willing to stay on indefinitely. 'Besides,' I added, 'that is a silly argument because you know very well that 95 percent of the people you hire are not ever going to be executive directors.' 'Yes,' he said, 'but there is always a possibility.'

"I went through all the nonsense about well, there are certain advantages to someone my age too. I have learned a certain amount about getting along with people and having judgment in certain situations. I'm not going to leave and go and have children.

"One of the things that has happened at this stage of my life is that I have found I'm much healthier. I don't get colds as often. For instance, I've been working at the same place for two years and I haven't been out for one day. I just feel exuberant."

INTERVIEW 2

"A woman is relegated to one corner, and if she tries to get out of that box, she has to really fight her way out. You're not considered a serious person if you're older."

These angry words were spoken by a woman who enjoyed the traditional roles of wife and mother and who has made a graceful transition to what the sociologists have termed "postparenthood." It is her work as a job counselor for older people that has made her painfully aware of prejudices against older people, especially older women, as workers. Struggling and often succeeding in finding jobs for women who are entering the marketplace for the first time when their children are grown, she has learned what a difficult transition many women must make. Her own menopause is a change she accepts with relative equanimity.

"About the time I began menopause I became a paid professional career counselor, and based on what my work has taught me, I urge every woman to get busy—from the age of twenty on.

"So much of what we call 'menopausal depression' is induced by the society in which we live. We are made to feel so depressed in so many ways, and it is so difficult for a woman who wants to get back to work or wants to go back to a career after she has raised a family. For those women who made separations and said, 'I will get my education, then I will get married and then I will raise a family and then go back and do this,' it becomes very difficult.

"In my work, I have encountered many older people looking for work, especially women, and I would say thousands are now returning to work after a life spent raising children. There is a feeling that has always been inculcated into women in our society that they are inferior, that they are very emotional, that they are not dependable, that they don't respond well to crises, that they don't make decisions—all that nonsense. This has made a very profound impression on a lot of women in my generation. I think that so many women in the younger generation are doing things in parallel fashions, which I think makes so much more sense. I'm sure many more people would do it if we had more adequate child care facilities available. I think it would be good if women really had outlets open to them all through their family-rearing years and all the other years when they are maturing, and had adequate vocational counseling so that they could begin to prepare themselves, even if they could only do it slowly and in a limited way. As it stands now, society is almost doing you a favor by letting you work. Some employers really feel like early Christian martyrs if they are asked to hire an older woman. A number of them say, 'Sure, we don't discriminate.' But I don't believe that there is really a deep-seated acceptance of the need to hire older women.

"Still, we've had good success in placing older women in jobs. One of the most gratifying things is that they acquire a feeling of aliveness and they can do something. You can really see it in the way they come in, the way they dress and walk, and the way they talk about themselves. There is a lot of excitement generated when someone values them enough to pay them for a job. This is really tremendous. In a sense, however, it is really pitiful that they should be so delighted with so little. I think women are beginning to realize that there is another world after family and children, and I'm not talking about death—I'm talking about living, really living.

"I worked until I had children. Work was something that I enjoyed and that I always had to do. For many years while I was married I did volunteer work. I then decided to go back and get a graduate degree.

I got a masters in human relations, the field I've always wanted to work in.

"It all depends on what interests you. There are marvelous jobs, very good pay in interesting fields, for example, for a good secretary. There is nothing to be ashamed of in being a good secretary. If you are smart enough, you can learn the business. I once worked as a secretary to a public relations director and that was absolutely smashing. I loved it.

"As far as menopause goes, I've been very fortunate: I feel fine physically and I've never gone through any depression or anything one learns from the myths. Menopause has not affected my sex life or my interest in sex. In addition, both my husband and I enjoy an active social life. We go to plays or concerts or go out to visit friends two or three times a week.

"At fifty-two or fifty-three my periods became less regular. Since I had always menstruated very regularly, even the shift of a day meant something serious—like pregnancy. I'd begun to have symptoms of menopause such as hot flashes and occasional palpitations, and my doctor suggested I try estrogen. I've been taking it for about five years in the lowest possible dosage and have not experienced any side effects. This has relieved the symptoms. My doctor, who is in favor of no medication at all unless indicated, encouraged me to call him whenever I felt anything irregular and suggested I try stopping the estrogen to see if the symptoms were still there. I've done this occasionally—this time for as long as six months—but the hot flashes have returned. It's discouraging. I still get occasional light periods, but they are almost nonexistent.

"I must admit that I looked forward to menopause with great eagerness at one time. I thought: Get all this crap out of the way. I have three children and had one abortion. I was always fearful I'd get pregnant. Also, I always thought menopause would give me a great deal of physical freedom, which didn't turn out to be the case. You are really not that much hampered by menstruation. I must say this whole thing is tied up with the process of getting older and knowing a definite phase of your life is over. Sometimes, rarely, I wish I could have another child. When I do, I think about my grandchildren. I adore children, and I think babies are the greatest thing in the world.

"The worst problems I had were episodes of heavy bleeding, when I thought I was hemorrhaging. It could be very embarrassing. I used to walk around with loads of tampons and sanitary napkins. I'd be standing in a counseling room with forty people and feel that something was dripping down. That happened very often, and the doctor thought he would have to do a D and C, to see what was happening. Several times it was scheduled and then the bleeding would stop. He would then call the surgery off. He doesn't believe in any unnecessary surgery.

"The doctor seemed to think it was related to having fibroids. But he said this happens to many women in menopause, and I know many women who have had the same experience. I felt anemic and took an iron supplement, which I still take once a day.

"Someone I know had told me about a product that I had never heard of before. It was a little cup that you insert and use like a tampon, but you can rinse it and use it over. I meant to ask my doctor about it but I forgot. My friend finds them really useful, and she bleeds a great deal and has had D and Cs. Heavy bleeding is a very common thing, evidently.

"Women friends have been very reassuring. We talk about symptoms that we have in common. I think we are much more open about talking about ourselves than men. We are never so frightened about a physical problem that we don't talk about it.

"Unless women are really incapacitated, this is the time that they should start doing the work that they always wanted to, if it's humanly possible. There are still many areas of interest that are open to women, and they should concentrate on them. This is their time."

INTERVIEW 3

"Menopause is not horrible. There's nothing horrible about it. It was a little bit annoying at that particular time—and that was that."

The speaker is a woman who is currently going through menopause. Even though she works in a health-related profession, she did not realize at first that the odd symptoms she has been experiencing were signs of menopause. She has adopted a kind of stiff upper lip attitude common to many active women who find that the challenge or distraction of work enables them to ignore physical discomforts. Her negative attitude toward having a Pap smear is especially interesting and disconcerting for someone supposedly more knowledgeable than average about health care. Many other women, it should be noted, similarly denied that they might have to face a serious physical problem by neglecting to have routine pelvic examinations or do breast self-examination.

"I have been around medicine for about thirty-five years—as a medical technician—so I did know what menopause was all about. However, when it happened to me, I didn't know it was happening, although I should have. But I'm a human being and I didn't stop to think.

"I kept waking up with night-sweats and at first thought that I was coming down with TB, because you start sweating that way. But still and all, I was all right in the daytime—I did my work and I thought, I can't possibly be coming down with anything. So finally it dawned on me; after that I didn't get excited or anything. I was about fifty then.

"At that time, I was living alone; my husband had been dead for two years. Sometimes I would get up, make myself something to eat, read the paper or listen to the radio, and then go back to bed. I never had trouble sleeping; I always had been pretty active and when nighttime came there was no keeping me up.

"It's difficult to say how long the flushes last because I can be in a sweat working around the house for an hour, and I am not certain if that's flushes. At night when I'm asleep I am not aware until I wake up. And then, of course, when you get out from under the covers you cool off. I found I was able to go back to sleep fairly easily.

"The night sweats lasted for about two years, not steadily—they could come months apart. I am not sure whether I still really have flushes or not. I may yell in the morning with the sun shining, 'It's too hot.' And yet I'll put on long sleeves for later. As far as sweating in bed, I haven't done that for about a year.

"My doctor gave me estrogen, which did help. It stopped the sweating at night. I took two or three shots of estrogen, I would say, once one month, then a month later, then not for a span of time. The last one made me puff up with water and then I started to bleed, so I took progesterone to try and counteract it.

"I've always had an irregular period, and I still stain during the month; but I'm not frightened because I know my hormones are mixed up.

"I stopped the hormone treatment myself. I didn't need it, and I didn't see any reason to take it. And whether in the future I will or not, I don't know. If I thought it would help or that I needed it, I would take it for as long as I needed it. And I wouldn't say it would cause cancer; I'm not concerned with that. The same as I don't want a Pap smear, because I don't feel I need one. There's time enough for that. You'll get warning. You would start bleeding or something like that. That's the only way they know. And as far as the breasts go—most women find lumps themselves, not the doctor. They feel something, or are taking a shower and are drying themselves and find a lump.

"Most of the symptoms of menopause, I think, are still up in the head and you just have to get it through your thick skull that you are not falling apart. I didn't find it disabling in any way. It just took me time until I finally figured it out. It didn't stop me from going anyplace or doing anything. If I go to bed and can't sleep, I watch the late show. I don't blame that on anything.

"My body feels the same, and I can do everything I did before. The heat is about the only thing I can say is different. I know some people say they turn red, but I haven't, and I haven't seen it happen to anybody else.

"A lot of people say they are nervous. I don't think I'm more nervous; I think I'm calm if I want to be unless I get picked on or something and then of course I probably am under tension. I think that a lot of stuff you read is baloney. Nervousness, depression, and anxiety don't come from menopause. They come from somewhere in the house or somebody in the house. A woman can be anxious when she's thirty years old. She could be crazy as a bedbug.

"I can't say that menopause makes you feel any different from any other time in your life. Circumstances around you may make a difference. Women eat too much because they have time on their hands and don't know what else to do. And it's not because they can't have children anymore. They're getting older, and they don't want any more kids. I don't think a man of fifty or sixty would want kids either. Women get fat because they're bored.

"Children never came along in my life, and I never bothered to find out why. It was just one of those things. If they had come along, I guess I would have enjoyed them; but I wasn't longing for one, like something that I had to have.

"I don't regret not having children. Actually, I don't feel that I'm alone or anything like that. I get along with most people. I share a house with a man I'm involved with, and I also have my animal companions. It would be difficult to lose them.

"Menopause doesn't have any effect on your sex life. Sex has nothing to do with the ability to reproduce. Women who complain that sex is different after menopause—that is an excuse. They don't want to be bothered. I don't want to be bothered if I'm dead tired, but it's because I'm just pooped out. I don't think it would be any different for a man either.

"Change of life does not have anything to do with your sexual drive. You do what you want in whatever way you want. I hold onto a lamp and swing. In other words, no holds barred.

"Maybe I'm not plagued, or wasn't plagued, with problems about menopause because until it dawned on me that this was what I was going through, I felt fine in the daytime and went to work. I don't think I missed a day's work in thirty years and I also kept house and cooked. I don't do quite as much now because my present house is bigger. Actually, I am happy about going through a change of life. No personal mess, no bother, tampons, and what-not.

"Menopause is nothing to be afraid of. No mystery. There are times in life when you have to go through the same sort of thing. It's like your period—you have to go through that—a week or whatever and it'll be over with. And that's the way it is with menopause. You have symptoms—heat or whatever you want to call it—but that's about all you feel. You are not supposed to get fat because of menopause and as far as I know you're not supposed to get nervous. I think I got over menopause nicely.

"As far as thinking you're old, I've got twenty years yet to go. I hope that as long as I live I will never have to be disabled or be put in a wheelchair. I would like to get about on my own, and I probably will. I'm pretty much of a jack-of-all-trades, so I don't think I'm going to fall apart. I am used to being active where other people sit down; maybe they have time to sit and think. I don't."

INTERVIEW 4

"All of a sudden, I began to realize that I had been asleep for years. I was changing and all kinds of thoughts came into my head at once."

Some women find the role of housewife and mother satisfying; here is one who did not. Whether it was baking cookies, going to PTA meetings, or chauffeuring her son to lessons, the daily round of activities of the suburban mother meant little but boredom to a woman who came to find that taking responsibility for her own life was exciting and a challenge.

"When I think of it now, I have walked through much of my life in a dream. I was married and lived in the suburbs, but I didn't belong to the superdomestic set; I didn't feel at home in it. After I suffered a severe but brief depression, I decided I had to get out and do something. I was in my late thirties. I started getting reinvolved in art, which I'd been interested in at college. I remember having the feeling that everybody else was doing something. Some of my friends who were working would say: 'You don't realize how lucky you are. You don't have to worry about bills, and you don't have to do this, and you don't have to do that.' It was true. But there were still things lacking.

"I was beginning to get energetic again, and I decided to take some courses at the university. Before this, I had accepted a passive child-wife role. I wouldn't go places without my husband. He probably wouldn't have minded, but I felt that he would. The idea of going out alone at night seemed strange to me. But I decided that I was going to take a course. And I went once a week and found it very exciting. It was the most important thing going on in my life at that time—which doesn't say much for my life, but it was the most intellectual stimulation I had. Meanwhile, I also started studying painting again. I studied with a very good teacher, just for fun. It was hard, but it sort of renewed me. I got much more interested in things, I made friends and, one piece at a time, my web started expanding.

"I don't think I went through menopause until I was about forty-seven, and I finished it about two years later—four years ago. As far as I was concerned, I didn't notice any real change. I felt very much alive at that period.

"I took none of the hormones, because I have a circulatory problem. Also, when I was about thirty-five my gynecologist gave me birth control pills. I immediately began to get headaches that woke me up at night, so she said, 'Stop, it's too risky.' For the same reason, my doctor advised me not to take estrogen. She said that the less you take, the better off you are.

"In my forties, I began to really want to do something. My husband always had his work, which absorbed him a great deal. He's also more of a solitary type, and was satisfied with the kind of life he led. I really liked to be out with people more, so I started working once a week with a friend who was a food stylist. But I didn't like it, so I went back to the hospital in which I had worked before I was married, and I got the best job I ever had. It was exciting, it was interesting, it was meaningful. They taught us psychiatry on the job. You had to know some basic psychiatry, but, more important, you had to relate well to people.

"When I look back on it, it was a rehabilitation for me. I liked the work, and the people were kind and close-knit; it was a team effort. We were a mixed bag, but were all very sensitive to each others' needs. It was the kind of place where, if you came in one day looking like you were worried or concerned, you'd find everybody ready to help you. And each contribution was individual; nobody else could make it. We got feedback in everything we did.

"I think, in some ways, my husband and I were drawing further apart, because my world was so different. I met a lot of new people. Suddenly I was getting more independent, and changing. I think I can really say that I woke up about that time.

"I can't tell you how this related to menopause. Here I was running around the place, doing all kinds of things. I don't know if I ever had any symptoms, except maybe an occasional hot flash. But they were so innocuous I didn't worry about them. I've never seen anybody turn red in the face. I've heard about it, but I've never seen it happen.

"At work I was encouraged to get out and do more things with my group. They wanted me to go places, to be freer, really. I felt that I couldn't or shouldn't because I was married. I had come from a generation that didn't do things without their husbands. I felt I should be at home. I think it was a very hard time. Both of us had a way of not communicating, which was bad. It was as if we were walking around a body in the living room, stepping over it and ignoring it.

"By now, I wanted more money, more autonomy, better hours, and all kinds of things, and I found my present job: I train and supervise occupational therapists who work with emotionally disturbed children.

"Eventually, my husband and I separated—I think because my son got very upset when he felt the coldness in the house. I had always thought I could cover up everything, but obviously I couldn't. So my husband moved out. Within the last year we have been getting along well. We really like each other. We're very good friends now. I think that there are certain needs that we still don't fulfill in one another, but we've known each other for so long that we're like blood relatives. You just can't walk away from it.

"I've thought of getting a divorce, but my husband doesn't want one. As for me, there's nobody I'm very interested in at this point in my life. I don't know what would happen if I fell in love with somebody, but right now, I can't envision that happening.

"It's lonesome. I feel that now I'm alone with myself in a way. I managed to maneuver it so that I could work and support myself, but now I've maneuvered myself back into this lonely position.

"I lost my mother last year—she had lived with me, but she was senile. My son is in college now, but he was never very companionable. He was always on the go, and I really wanted him to be independent.

"I've been going to school at night for some time. I now have my B.S. in psychology, and I have almost half of my master's. That's going to take a long time, and I'm not even sure that I want it.

"Right now, if I had my druthers, and enough money, I don't think I would work. I'd travel, I'd stay home—all these things that I was never interested in before and my husband was interested in. Now I'd like to be digging in the garden, and I've started gardening for the first time in my life. I used to love the city; now I love the country. I've just grown up late. I'm tired of working, but I don't have a choice. I'm paying a lot of bills.

"I did go to Europe, five years ago, and I went alone. I got the Eurailpass—I just took off—and I loved it. I didn't feel lonely. I've taken a few cruises. I would rather have company on those, but I never have had, and I've never missed it as much as I thought I might. I don't like female company very much. I can't see going with a group of women.

"I'd be interested in meeting a man. I'm not necessarily sure about the sexual thing. But I would like stimulating companionship, and I really miss the security.

"I'm in a funny position right now. In one way, my husband's still very much in my life, but I don't think that I'm much in his. Actually, I think that's the way it's always been. He's off and doing his own thing, whatever it may be. He's independent and very energetic and does whatever he wants. I would really like to live a less solitary life."

INTERVIEW 5

"I was so damn tired all the time. Even the gals in the office noticed it. I was not myself. I was feeling rotten, and I finally quit my job."

At age forty-nine, this mother of four had a hysterectomy to remove fibroid tumors, which were causing her to hemorrhage. Her doctor chose that occasion to remove her ovaries, giving no medical explanation for why that was necessary. (It may or may not have been, but without interviewing the doctor it would be impossible to know.) She had a sudden menopause as the result of surgery and has been taking estrogen for ten years. With all of her physical problems, she still feels fortunate to have a mutually loving relationship with her husband.

"I was never oriented toward getting a job. I've only worked four years in my whole married existence, starting about two or three years before my menopause when I was about forty-six. I was always interested in anything to do with medicine. I was always a frustrated nurse, so I found myself looking in the hospital/health fields. And I found a marvelous job, as it happened, working for the head of pediatrics at the hospital nearby. It was a very exciting office. I was the departmental secretary, and I learned my job in a hurry. It was very busy. There was no time to breathe, and this was my first job. I was a wreck. I went every morning, thinking I couldn't possibly do a good job. I also went thinking, 'I've lived this really kind of sheltered existence, where I've always been my own boss. I don't like the idea of people telling me what to do.' It was a different thing. I wasn't the mother or the boss; I was suddenly being told, you do this, you do that.

"I worked there for two years, and just before I left, I was becoming tired. Not just from doing the work, but feeling lousy all the time. I was beginning to have fewer periods. I had always been regular before that, extremely regular. Every twenty-eight or twenty-nine days, it would last three or four days, and no problem. I suddenly started missing a few, feeling kind of funny.

"I also had headaches, and I was really upset because I wanted to feel good. I noticed I was really cranky. Strange, funny feelings. When I hear people who have been on dope describe withdrawal, it sounds like the same strange sensations in the arms and legs. It would wake me up at night. It was like someone was draining all the blood out of me. When I went to the gynecologist, she said that there were women who had these curious symptoms, which they were never able to do anything about. But doctors have heard of them.

"Also at that time, just before I stopped working, I had trouble with my breasts. My nipples started bleeding one night. It was really scary because I had never had any problems before. The first thing you think of is that you must have cancer. A surgeon at the hospital where I was working did a biopsy. I was just in the hospital overnight, and he showed me the actual lab report on the day I came back to work; he said he just wanted me to see it so I would believe it. It was a benign polyp.

"At the same time, I kept thinking in the back of my mind, 'This was just one; maybe I'll have trouble with the other. Maybe it won't be a polyp.' You do think of that sort of thing, naturally. But I never spent a lot of time worrying. I do remember saying to my doctor, though, 'What if you send the biopsy out while I'm in surgery and you find that I have cancer, what will you do? I would want you to wake me up and talk to me about it. I don't want to wake up and find myself without a bosom.' He said he would not do anything at the time, and would certainly discuss it with me. It would naturally be a terribly traumatic thing, but I think that I would manage it, as bad as I thought it would look to me—like being a little girl again.

"I remember the time of my hysterectomy. I had a hemorrhage. I went to the doctor in the afternoon, and he gave me an injection. He said that if he gave it to me, it might help. When he examined me, he said I probably had a fibroid tumor and would probably have to have a hysterectomy.

"I knew that I probably would have to have a hysterectomy; but that didn't really bother me. I have never been uncomfortable in hospitals. If I go to a hospital, I have to know everything that's going to happen. I feel better knowing. My own doctor won't answer any questions on his own. You have to ask him.

"They knew it was a fibroid tumor. The doctor was a conservative guy, and he said to me that I had to have surgery. I was so sick I didn't give a damn at that point anyway. I was forty-nine, and he said there was no point in keeping my ovaries: 'We might as well take the whole business out.' And I said, 'Of course, what do I need my ovaries for?' After it was all over, it was really funny, he said, 'You know, I took out your appendix, too. It was right next door.'

"I had a perfectly normal recuperation, except that I was plunged into menopause.

"Because I had all these kinds of crazy pains, my doctor sent me to an osteopath. They stuck me in the hospital and put me through all these horrible crazy tests. And I also had a psychiatrist talking to me for two hours. He said, 'You don't have to worry, because I could swear it's not a psychological thing with you. You're going through what a lot of women go through during menopause, and it will gradually lessen. Because you're so involved with it, this has added a little bit to your condition, but we don't consider it psychological.' You always feel angry when they say its psychosomatic, when you're feeling lousy. But everything adds to everything. And in the family there were problems, tensions I felt that may have been part of it.

"During menopause, there were maybe one or two nights that I had what you call sweats, but I never recall waking up in sweats. I did have flashes off and on during the day. My face got red; it would absolutely burn up. But very rarely—this was not a big thing with me. Everybody I've spoken to has had this problem, and it can be very embarrassing. Once I had a hot flash after a doctor's examination. I suddenly became hot, and he was standing right behind me. I was just so uncomfortable. I said, 'Well, you can see that I'm having a hot flash right now.' It was just so nauseating. He said, 'Well, it must be awful for people who get sweaty, and it's embarrassing.' Well, what do you say, 'Pardon me, I'm just having a hot flash'?

"Three or four months after surgery my doctor put me on estrogen. I didn't ask for it. I figured I was feeling lousy because of surgery. I started taking it when I began to get back my strength. I still felt strange, and my bones ached; it was driving me bananas. My doctor spoke to me about the hormones. I went back to the gynecologist about a month or so after I came home from the hospital. The first time he just gave me an internal examination. The next time I sat and talked with him for a while because I was having these weird feelings. I told him that my own doctor had suggested taking estrogen. He said, 'He's absolutely right.' So I started taking it. I'm going to be fifty-nine now.

"I took myself off it a couple of months ago. It didn't seem to be doing me that much good. There was all this publicity about estrogen, though I knew I didn't have to worry about cervical cancer. I didn't feel better or worse or anything. But I kept myself off for a couple of months, and I don't know whether it was psychological or not, but I wasn't feeling that good. And I did have a hot flash. So I put myself right on again. I certainly don't want to worry about having to go through hot flashes. I'm uncomfortable enough.

"My sex life hasn't changed since surgery. I must say I have no problems there whatsoever. With the pains in my muscles and the pains in my bones, we try all kinds of positions. I never even thought about that in relation to my hysterectomy. It does take time for you to get back, you feel so rotten. It's like after you have a child, and it takes time for you to feel good down there.

"My friends asked several hundred questions after my hysterectomy. I was the first among them to become pregnant, to have an abortion, and to have a hysterectomy, so I was the one they came to as the woman of experience. They also sort of expected that this could happen. It wasn't as though you were having a hysterectomy in your twenties and thirties. At this time in life it wasn't so terrible, if you had your family and you expected it. I had no feeling that this was a hysterectomy done quickly and with no thought, to make money or just a convenience for the doctor. My own doctor is extremely conservative, and before he thinks of surgery you go through all kinds of tests.

"Of course, all this time I was having a lot of support from my husband. We are very lucky. We're very happy together, and we look forward to seeing each other, being with each other. So I had that kind of support, and I have kids who are very close and good and fun. So that part of it was very good.

"I have never felt great, but I don't think this has anything to do with menopause. I haven't *really* felt good since before my hysterectomy. I put on a great big act and I do everything, and I look pretty good, so I get absolutely no sympathy; then again, I wouldn't want them to say, 'Oh, you look horrible.' I have some kind of muscular/skeletal problem, but, thank God, I don't have any muscle disease that they can find. I have good days and bad days. When I had trouble with my tear ducts, the eye doctor said to me, 'I'm not the least bit surprised that you're having this because this has something to do with muscles.'

"But with all that, I don't feel too badly, either. I just don't feel as comfortable as I'd like to feel.

"I notice, since our kids have left us, my husband and I are closer in a different way. You start living a different kind of life after the kids leave; you start again. If you've been fortunate enough like us to have really loved one another and enjoyed each other and you have a good sense of humor—a sense of saneness about everything—and you also know that there are always going to be things that you're going to disagree about, then things are prime and you can manage to enjoy each other and keep everything together. It is not always easy, naturally. But we are fortunate in that respect.

"I plan to start doing some volunteer work now that my husband is retired and things are quieter. For a while, I did some work at the hospital. Just going in and talking to patients. I'm not too bright, but I'm awfully good at this sort of thing, but it took too much out of me.

"I wish I could still play tennis. Just the other day, I tried for awhile, but I couldn't move around. I felt weak, and I made an appointment with the doctor, because I knew he would have to give me an injection. That irritates me. But there are other things I can do, so I'm not gonna be a nut about it.

"I enjoy writing. I'm the kind of person who watches people. I've jotted down things about this one and that one, and I decided that I'd like to write stories about the people I've observed.

"I also want to do a little bit of traveling. We have two kids on the West Coast, so we want to take some time off, now that my husband doesn't have to worry about getting back.

"It's a different feeling. We're really free. Our children's lives are really their own responsibility. I'm glad to see them doing well, and I'm happy for them.

"You feel the way you did before you had children, except that you do have a family. And you're not physically the same. I can remember my mother saying, 'The heat—I just can't stand it.' She was knocked out. And I remember saying to myself, 'What's she talking about?' Now I do the same thing myself. The sun bothers me. And I think that I couldn't possibly have related to that in my twenties or thirties. You feel OK, but not great. Some days, I can't get out of bed; I can't bend over; I can't clench my fists. Well, it's not such a big thing, but it's different. You slow down just a little bit. But I can't say that I have too many complaints. I can get up; I can use my mind and body."

INTERVIEW 6

"My husband was aware that something was wrong. I was awfully hard to get along with. Before I realized what it was, I couldn't understand what was the matter with me. I don't know how he ever stood it. He's most patient."

Like so many women in her age group, the woman who spoke these words had never discussed menopause with anyone—not her mother or her sister or a close friend; and like many others she was not aware for some time that the feelings and changes she was experiencing were the result of a natural process.

"It bothers me when I think how old I am, but what can you do about it anyway? I think of the things that I could do, and I think, I can't do that. Nobody would want anybody fifty-seven to get a job or go through nursing school or things like that. Things that I haven't done, that I think, 'Gee, I should have done this years ago.' I always wanted to go to nursing school, for example, but they probably wouldn't take me now.

"I didn't work while I was raising my children. In fact, I was offered a job and refused. My husband's office did not want to bring in any more new people, and they tried to get the wives to take the clerical jobs. But I decided that I wanted to raise my own children. When the youngest was in the fifth grade, they were all in school all day, and my husband started traveling almost half the time. I began to get terribly depressed. In fact, I think I was almost suicidal, I was so depressed. And it looked as if it was going to be the same the next year. I took myself in hand and decided that I had to do something. I felt that I had no experience, but I felt I had to do something. I was looking through the paper one Sunday, more or less as a lark, and I saw a part-time job advertised, which I thought I could fill. As a lark I went down and applied for it, and no one was more surprised than I when I was offered the job. I took it, and I was there for fourteen years.

"I didn't realize I was going through menopause until there was quite a space between my periods. I had also been irregular when I was a teen-ager. I used to become very ill and had terrible cramps. The same thing happened when I started to go into menopause. My period became as irregular as it had before. And it lengthened out. I can't say when it really started. All of a sudden, it would be three months. And then, all of a sudden, one day, I realized that it had been over a year. And then, of course, I started having the hot flashes. I felt like a teen-ager, because of the terrible cramps.

"I was in my mid-forties, I can't say what age exactly, but I think it was fairly early. I have a friend, for instance, who's the same age as I am. And I know that, as of three years ago, she was still as regular as clockwork.

"It annoyed me that I was feeling this way again. And I felt that I couldn't plan ahead because I never knew when I would start feeling miserable.

"It was when my period was coming every three months that I started having hot flashes. They were very distressing. I had them mostly at night, not too much during the day. It might happen several times during one night. Oh, it was terrible. It's a most unpleasant feeling. I would have to get up because I would be drenched. I think, actually, I got up before I had to, to keep the sheets from getting wet.

"It would happen only once in awhile during the day. I felt very lucky about that. I would think that during the day it could be very embarrassing—when you're in company, and suddenly you're in this terrible sweat. If it had ever happened in public with my husband, I think that I would have died. Because he would have come right out and said something, or made some remarks.

"I was very disagreeable. No matter what people wanted to do,

I wouldn't want to do it. I would complain bitterly and would be very nasty. My husband would say, "Why do you do things like that?" And I really wouldn't know. I felt like a fool. But I kept on doing it. This was before I became aware that I was going through menopause. I guess I wasn't expecting it at so early an age. This lasted for three or four years. I think it was hard for him. When I started having the irregular periods and the hot flashes, it became obvious what it was and this made it easier for both of us to cope with.

"I finally went to my family physician, mostly about the hot flashes. And I am very glad now that he didn't want to do anything about them, like give me hormones. The medications these days are so strong that I'm afraid to take anything. I asked him how long this was going to go on. He was very understanding, and said that there are women who are seventy-five who are having it. I figured that I would never live through it. Thirty more years! It actually lasted only a couple of years. It seemed longer, but I don't think it was.

"I don't think that it bothered me when I was at work. I didn't have the moodiness when I was at work. And the hot flashes were really not that much during the day. So I really don't think that it affected my work at all. It also didn't affect my sex life at all.

"I never really discussed menopause very much with anyone. I don't think that I had any really close friends at that time. We had moved around so much, and most of the friends we had were people that my husband worked with. I never really got friendly with any of their wives. My mother wasn't much help, because she had a different experience. She had a very serious operation at about the time when she would have had menopause, and according to the doctors this should have had no effect at all. But after she recovered from the operation, she never had any more menstruation, just never went through any of this.

"She never talked to me about menopause before it happened to me. Mother was not one to do that at all. She also hadn't prepared me for menstruation. She didn't tell me anything she didn't have to tell me.

"I don't think anybody told me any terrible stories about menopause. I really didn't know what to expect. While it was going on, I read some books that were sort of frightening. Things weren't as bad as, in some cases, the books made them seem, so in that way I was a little encouraged.

"I do resent the fact that I can't have any more children. I think that I would like to, though my husband wouldn't. He thought that starting again with a baby was crazy. He was probably right.

"I was working part time when my last child got married and left home, and at that time my husband was very ill. So I never had the useless feeling some women talk about. I really was useful. And then, a year later, my sister had some serious problems and came to stay with me for awhile. The next year there was a sick relative. I was involved with things of that sort, on top of working.

"I quit my job five years ago. Not until last year did I feel that I would like to start looking for a part-time job. I guess I really want something to do. I was kind of tired of working when I quit. I thought I would get tired of loafing right away, but I didn't. I was very happy not being at work for awhile. Now I think I do want to go back to work. I don't want to go through the same thing I did when I was younger and got so depressed."

INTERVIEW 7

"I very naïvely thought, until not too many years ago, that your sexual appetite, desires, reactions, and feelings just stopped when you had menopause. Isn't that crazy?"

Here is another woman who has suffered from ignorance of her own physiology and psychology—and from the veil that, until recently, our society threw over anything sexual. If women realized that they were full sexual beings and would continue being so until they died, would they plan their lives differently?

"I think that one's female life has a lot to do with how one feels about menopause. I am sixty-one and my mother was forty when I was born, so hers was a generation when parents' attitudes about what they told their children were different from what they are now. I did have loving and marvelous parents, but because of the time when I grew up and reached puberty, there wasn't a great deal of discussion. It didn't come as a total shock, but discussion of sexual matters was just not done. My mother told me very simply about a menstrual period—what it was, and that it would come about. I don't remember feeling any shock or displeasure. Luckily she told me in time, because

I didn't menstruate until a little bit later than average. I think I was fourteen. It was a slow process. My period was very spotty; there would be a long time and then another period.

"I had a very agonizing time in my adolescence. Even up until I was married, I had the most ghastly cramps. It must be what many women have in childbirth. It was so awful, I would practically faint. I think a lot of that is psychological, which has no bearing, because it felt real. The pain was so terrible that I would have to lie flat on the floor, and perspiration would just stream off my face. It was absolutely agonizing. It wasn't every month or all the time, but my mother and father took me to a doctor for a whole series of tests, to see if there was an endocrine imbalance in my system. It turned out not to be organic at all. The pain went on through graduate school, but it wasn't so bad then or while I was working. I was too busy to think about it; I was being a single, independent woman. In fact, nothing of that nature ever happened again, either in my married life or after.

"I wasn't married until I was thirty-one. I had a couple of engagements, but they didn't work out. I went to college and to graduate school, and then worked. Then I met my husband, and very quickly decided that this was the one. We were married in just a few short months. He was a good deal older than I. He had also never been married before. We very much wanted and intended to have children, but we went about it rather planfully. My first child wasn't born until I was thirty-three. The next was two-and-one-half years later. My third and last child was born when I was forty—she wasn't planned!

"At that time there wasn't any dilemma in my mind about whether or not to have children. Because I'd been an only child, I definitely didn't want to produce an only child. So it was all planned and happy —I anticipated it and it was all extremely healthy. I had not read about the possibiilty of Mongolism and had not thought about it, so I approached my pregnancies with no apprehension. I felt healthy and I was active, so there was no reason to worry. All three pregnancies were normal, and I don't remember any discomfort.

"In fact, giving birth to my first child was the most fulfilling experience I ever had in my life. It was my experience, somehow, and I'm not sure I would have wanted my husband involved in it. I just wanted to do it myself. Emotionally, I wouldn't want any distracting things. To produce a child is totally creative. I remember my first child's birth very vividly as the highlight of my whole life! It was so wonderful an experience that I don't even remember any agony. In fact, I remember enormous joy, just being part of the human race, being a woman and able to do what a man cannot do—a man cannot carry a baby and give birth to it. It's too bad; I feel rather sorry for men, I really do! Being a woman has never seemed to be my problem.

"And because I was older when I got married, I didn't go through what a lot of women of this generation are going through. I'd had about five or six years of being a professional woman, having a job I enjoyed doing, and being on my own. When I left it to be a wife and mother I saw that as the next chapter, not as being deprived of something. I don't remember any displeasure about any of it, I mean *real* displeasure. I just sort of went about it; it was part of having the children. Having children was part of being married, so it was a very interesting thing. I thoroughly enjoyed it, and I didn't feel put-upon. My husband was marvelous, so we had a real partnership, and we really shared the whole experience.

"Although I didn't have a job, I kept active the whole time, in a rather limited way, in civic things. I served on committees and boards. Only now that I have been working again for five years am I beginning to miss having a career.

"I began to think about menopause in my forties, not in a worrisome way, but because my contemporaries were talking about 'to take hormones or not to take hormones.' They're still discussing that. I've had doctors all along who weren't extremists in any way. So I wasn't exposed to any experiments or medications that had never been really proven. My doctor never suggested taking estrogen. He believed that, if I appeared healthy, there was no reason to give me anything. Yet I think I probably asked him. I had been reading all the advertisements and looking at my friends, whose complexions are really heavenly; you *can* see a difference. I'm not withered, but some women my age do have a much more beautiful, younger-looking skin. Maybe they *do* take hormones, maybe they don't. I've never had any kind of medication during menopause, and I've never had any complaint.

"My mother never talked to me about menopause. I knew from the textbooks what it was, and yet I didn't know quite what the symptoms were or just how it might come about. What I imagined was that, finally, your ovaries just didn't have to expel that lining regularly anymore, so they just sort of dried up. I really imagined this until I'd been to my gynecologist. It happened when I was fifty-three or fifty-four. Some of the symptoms were like a hemorrhaging. I went to the doctor and said 'My goodness, I used up all my tampons. What's happening?' I thought I was drying up, because my periods were getting less regular.

"I wasn't having any sexual intercourse by then, because my husband had long been dead. He died of a heart attack when the children were very young. We'd been married eleven years. That was the only sexual life I'd had, for which I'm very sad now, because that's when I was really in full flower. There was never any distaste, but it takes a long time, at least for a person of my temperament and background, to become receptive and enjoy it in the way it should be enjoyed. I was just at the point where that would probably have been happening in a very pleasurable way. All that came to an end abruptly, and I went into a very extreme depression.

"Fortunately, I had very *good* psychiatric care when this happened. For two months I was in a psychiatric hospital having a series of shock treatments, and then home for two months. That hadn't quite done the trick so I had to go back and have another series. When I came out I did very well, and I have ever since.

"At the beginning of menopause my periods got farther apart. I would skip. Instead of three or four or five weeks, it would be maybe eight weeks. And there was less of a flow. Since I was going to my gynecologist anyway, I didn't have to rush to the doctor thinking, 'Oh my gosh, am I having menopause?' or anything like that. I had security in the fact that every year I went for a complete physical. The doctor always asked me all the questions, and I always gave him all the answers.

"At the beginning I thought, 'Oh, this is wonderful; it will get less and less and that's it.' I didn't feel emotionally upset, and I wasn't having any other symptoms. The next thing that happened was the hemorrhaging, which I went to the doctor about. The only other symptom, which seemed to come later, was sweating in the night. I can remember waking up. It didn't disturb me very much—I didn't even have to change my nightgown—but I think that I must have told the doctor about it. It didn't bother me that I was going through menopause. I thought it was perfectly natural, and about time.

"I think, if you have a husband, menopause makes a difference. If you are married, there is always the feeling, 'Thank God, that's all over with now. I don't have to use the pill or the diaphragm.' But I had nothing to think about. I wasn't in love; I didn't really have any suitors; I didn't care for anyone. I guess I'm just one of those people who has one man. I don't make myself available, although I miss a man horribly; and at first I thought I would like to be remarried. I don't know what I want now, but it's very unsatisfactory to be a single person. I just think nature decreed that there be two people. I don't think there's any substitute for a man.

"Because you just don't see or hear about old people making love, I had no way of knowing whether people make love when they're old. I'm a very private person, and I don't look into other people's business. I've heard stories about strongly sexed older women—but I thought they were *very* unusual. I was all wrong! I have these feelings inside—and I feel deprived. But now it's too late. I can't do anything about it.

"In general, my attitude about menopause was that it was nothing to be afraid of; it was a natural part of life. Every female went through it. And if it was a part of life, there was nothing abnormal about it."

RESOURCE DIRECTORY

Although almost everything concerning menopause was considered for inclusion in this directory, we have tried to select only the most important, the most comprehensive, and sometimes the most innovative resources for the older woman.

When books are available in both hardcover and soft, only the paperback price is given. All listings have been verified by phone or mail.

HEALTH RESOURCES

Women's Health Centers

The following listings and descriptions of women's health centers cannot claim to be complete. Every day there seem to be more and more women interested in the women's health movement, and new centers spring up constantly.

We were told repeatedly by the health centers that they had some older women among their clientele but were eager to have more. Many health centers want or are just beginning to plan programs for older women. Those centers marked with an asterisk will offer menopause discussion groups if there is enough interest.

Reach for Recovery

Reach for Recovery is a rehabilitative program for women who have had breast surgery. Trained volunteers who have successfully adjusted to their own mastectomies visit patients who are recovering to provide reassurance and to distribute a helpful kit. Reach for Recovery also holds open forums on mastectomy and accompanies patients for the fitting of their first prosthesis. For information, contact your local branch of the American Cancer Society.

CALIFORNIA

Berkeley Women's Health Collective
2908 Ellsworth St.
Berkeley, Calif.   94705
(415) 843-6194

These women have an active program for older women—the Older Women's Function Group—which runs menopause rap sessions, lectures, self-help groups, and an open house once a month to attract new members. Fees are based on a sliding scale, with women paying only what they can afford.

Feminist Women's Health Center*
2930 McClure
Oakland, Calif.   94609
(415) 444-5676

This center offers gynecological care: pelvic exam, Pap test, and breast exam. Available on a rental basis is a videotape of women discussing their mastectomy experiences. Fees are on a sliding scale.

Feminist Women's Health Center*
1112 South Crenshaw Blvd.
Los Angeles, Calif.   90019
(213) 936-7219

This center offers basic gynecological care, with fees based on a sliding scale. A group at FWHC is currently working on a book about the mystique of the health care system as it affects women.

Feminist Women's Health Center
429 S. Sycamore St.
Santa Ana, Calif. 92701
(714) 547-0327

This center runs Well Women Clinics, which offer basic gynecological care. Fees are moderate.

San Francisco Women's Health Center
3789 24th St.
San Francisco, Calif. 94116

This health center holds menopause discussion groups in four-session series. Weekly meetings cover physiology, symptoms, treatment, nutrition, and exercise. Groups are kept small and attempt to be supportive.

Santa Cruz Women's Health Center*
250 Locust St.
Santa Cruz, Calif. 95606
(408) 427-3500

The women here would like more middle-aged women to use the services of their center, which include self-help groups, doctor referrals, and a library. Fees are low to moderate.

Womancare
1050 Garnet
San Diego, Calif. 92109
(714) 488-7591

Womancare is a group that offers general gynecological care for women, and it encourages older women to use the center. Self-help groups for middle-aged women have been offered and will continue to be, if there is enough interest. Fees are based on a sliding scale and there is a library available.

COLORADO

Women's Health Service Clinic of Colorado Springs
1703 N. Weber
Colorado Spring, Colo.   80907
(303) 471-9492

This feminist-oriented service is currently planning to offer menopause discussion groups. Their clinic provides basic gynecological care and sponsors sexual therapy groups. Instruction in self-examination is available.

CONNECTICUT

Women's Health Services, Inc.
19 Edwards St.
New Haven, Conn.   06511
(203) 777-4781

Women's Health Services offers pregnancy testing, abortions, and doctor referrals. Women's Health Education, a study/research group, which is a division of Women's Health Services, has offered lectures on menopause.

DISTRICT OF COLUMBIA

Women's Medical Center
1712 I St.
Washington, D.C.   20006
(202) 298-9227

This center has organized one of the most comprehensive menopause programs in the country. Susan McCarter, R.N., is in charge of the services, which include counseling, gynecological clinic, mutual support groups that can be held in the community, and a menopause bibliography and various pamphlets. Susan McCarter will speak to women's groups and is eager to talk to anyone who is working in this area.

FLORIDA

Feminist Women's Health Center*
1017 Thomasville Rd.
Tallahassee, Fla. 32303
(904) 224-9600

The Feminist Women's Health Center runs a Well Women Gynecology Clinic for women of all ages. It is financed from donations and from the moderate fees received from its patients. There is a small library.

Women's Health Center
805 Fourth Ave. S.W.
Gainsville, Fla. 32601
(904) 377-5055

The women who run this center consider a menopausal woman to be a well woman. The medical part of their program is called "The Well Woman Clinic." It offers basic gynecological care, with fees based on a sliding scale. The center has self-help groups and has created a slide presentation about self-help. There is a library with a Xerox machine, where you may read and do research. A menopause fact sheet is available upon request.

ILLINOIS

HERS
2748 N. Lincoln
Chicago, Ill. 60614
(312) 528-2736

HERS is an acronym for Health Evaluation Referral Service. It can give you names and evaluations of doctors and feminist therapists. Also, HERS runs menopause discussion groups and distributes informational literature about menopause.

Suburban Women's Health Center
837 S. Westmore
Lombard, Ill. 60148
(312) 495-9330

Providing education and information about women's health care is an important function of the Suburban Women's Health Center. It publishes a menopause pamphlet and provides doctor referrals. Individual counseling is available at moderate fees.

IOWA

The Emma Goldman Clinic for Women*
715 North Dodge
Iowa City, Iowa 52240
(319) 337-2111

The women at Emma Goldman are working on a book about herbal healing, which will include a chapter on menopause. Basic gynecological care is offered at the clinic, as well as self-help groups. There are massage classes, and a masseuse is available. The clinic also has a library. Fees are computed on a sliding scale.

Women's Community Health Center
819 Lincoln Way
Ames, Iowa 50010
(515) 232-9078

This women's health center would particularly like to reach out to middle-aged women. It has held both menopause discussion groups and self-help groups for older women. Other services include doctor referrals, a Well Women Gynecology Clinic, and a library. Women are permitted to pay 50 or 75 percent of the fee if they are unable to pay the full amount.

RESOURCE DIRECTORY | 207

LOUISIANA

Delta Women's Clinic
1406 St. Charles Ave.
New Orleans, La.   70130
(504) 581-2288

Delta Women's Clinic is primarily an abortion clinic. However, it serves many middle-aged women with abortion and sterilization services and has a complete community referral service, a library, a speakers' bureau, Gestalt therapy groups, and student fieldwork placement programs for women who are attending college.

MAINE

Women's Center of Portland
193 Middle St.
Portland, Me.   04111
(207) 774-6071

There is no longer a women's health center in Maine. The Women's Center, however, will try to help you with doctor referrals. These women can also provide divorce counseling and divorce discussion groups.

MASSACHUSETTS

Somerville Women's Health Project
326 Somerville Ave.
Somerville, Mass.   02143
(617) 666-5290

This free clinic has been in existence for five years. Last year it sponsored a menopause group led by a mental health professional and a woman who had experienced menopause. The group ran successfully for eight months and the center is interested in helping to form another such information/support/discussion group. Clinic hours are at night and basic gynecological care is offered. The clinic is staffed by volunteer doctors and nurses. Patient-advocates are a feature of the medical program.

Women's Community Health Center, Inc.
137 Hampshire St.
Cambridge, Mass. 02139
(617) 547-2302

This group runs four-week special interest groups (some have been on menopause). All groups begin with a slide show, which is an introduction to self-help and women's health care.

MICHIGAN

Feminist Women's Health Center
2445 W. 8 Mile Rd.
Detroit, Mich. 48203
(313) 892-7790

This is primarily an abortion facility, but it will make doctor referrals for older women.

MINNESOTA

Elizabeth Blackwell Women's Health Center*
200 S. 5th St.
Minneapolis, Minn. 55454
(612) 335-7669

This center has a library, a speakers' bureau, and a health care referral service, and offers a general eight-week class in women's health.

MISSOURI

The Women's Self-Help Center
8129 Delmar St., Room 204
St. Louis, Mo. 63130
(314) 862-2202

This new center does not yet offer the full range of programs that are being planned. At present, it offers abortions and doctor referrals. The Women's Self-Help Center would like to work with someone interested in running menopause-discussion groups.

NEW MEXICO

Women's Health Services
700 Franklin St.
Sante Fe, N. Mex. 87501
(505) 988-2660

As we go to press, Women's Health Services claims to have the only woman doctor in Santa Fe. Working within a small budget, this center is able to offer a wide range of services: basic gynecological care, counseling, sex therapy groups, self-help groups, a lending library, and a general medical clinic. It is a nonprofit organization with fees based on a sliding scale.

NEW YORK

Eastern Women's Center
14 E. 60th St.
New York, N.Y. 10022
(212) 832-0033   (24-hour emergency number: 832-0099)

In conjunction with the American Cancer Society, the Eastern Women's Center provides free Pap tests. The center does complete gynecological examinations, which include a short film on Pap smears and breast exams.

210 | RESOURCE DIRECTORY

It has a free speakers' bureau and conducts sexuality courses, which are open to men and women. This center also provides abortions.

Recently Dr. Helen DeRosis and Victoria Pellegrino, authors of *The Book of Hope: How Women Can Overcome Depression*, held seminars here on "Overcoming Depression and Building Self-Esteem," which proved to be so popular that they are now held weekly.

St. Marks Clinic
44 St. Marks Place
New York, N.Y. 10003
(212) 533-9500

St. Marks is a small community-based, ambulatory-care facility. It has a special women's night from 5:00 to 10:00 P.M. on Tuesdays, staffed exclusively by women, usually a doctor and a paramedic. This clinic tries to respond to the needs and concerns of women whose problems are often ignored by the health care system—for example, older women and lesbians. Unlike many other clinics, it does not handle birth control. St. Marks welcomes middle-aged patients. The fee is $5 per visit plus the cost of lab tests and medication. Patients who cannot afford the cost of a visit are never refused.

The 78th Street Health Center
1120 Lexington Ave.
New York, N.Y. 10021
(212) 861-0429

This three-year-old center provides basic gynecological care for all women, including older women. The fees ($35 for basic visit) are higher than those listed for most health centers, but this organization is highly rated by other feminist groups.

The center has one very special feature—a "change of persona" program for women who want to change their sex. Before a woman is accepted into the program, she must undergo an extensive consultation and exam. Then a long-range plan for the change is drawn up. Intense training in personality change is offered for those women who feel deeply dissatisfied with their sexual identity.

OREGON

The Women's Health Clinic*
4160 S.E. Division
Portland, Ore. 97202
(503) 234-9774

The Women's Health Clinic is a free clinic, staffed by paramedics, nurses, medical students, and lab technicians. It has been functioning in Portland since 1971. It's services include gynecological exams, doctor referrals, and counseling.

PENNSYLVANIA

Elizabeth Blackwell Health Center for Women
112 South 16th St.
Philadelphia, Pa. 19102
(215) 563-7577

This center sees older women in its gynecology service and occasionally has a free cancer screening program. A menopause workshop for women over forty is offered. The workshop begins with factual information on menopause and women's health. Thereafter, the group is left on its own to share feelings and to lend support-to its members.

CHOICE
1501 Cherry St.
Philadelphia, Pa. 19102
(215) 567-7392   (Hot line: 567-2904)

CHOICE describes itself as a nonprofit consumer-advocate organization concerned with reproductive health care for women. The staff will try to answer any questions women have concerning health care, and they can make doctor referrals. In the area of women's sexuality, CHOICE has been running workshops designed as educational-enrichment experiences rather than discussions of sexual mechanics.

One of CHOICE's staff members, Bobbie Whitney, has been doing research about menopause and is eager to speak to women about their experiences.

UTAH

Feminist Women's Health Center*
363 E. 6th St.
Salt Lake City, Utah   84404
(801) 328-3032

This center, staffed primarily by volunteers, offers basic gynecological care. There is a film on mastectomy available for interested women's groups.

VERMONT

Southern Vermont Women's Health Center*
18 N. Main St.
Rutland, Vt.   16501
(802) 775-1056

With many middle-aged women among its clientele, this center provides annual gynecological exams. The center is a nonprofit corporation, run as a collective, with fees on a sliding scale. Short-term counseling, related to health or sexuality, is available.

The Vermont Women's Health Center
Box 29, 158 Bark St.
Burlington, Vt.   05401

Since 1972, the VWHC has been helping women with their medical problems. The health center is run as a collective and offers a wide range of services for older women including counseling, gynecological exams, and programs on recovery from hysterectomy and mastectomy. One of the top priorities is to encourage older women to use the center, and it would like to organize a self-help group for older women.

WASHINGTON

Aradia Clinic
4224 University Way, N.E.
Seattle, Wash. 98105

Aradia does not yet have specific services for older women. It does, however, offer general gynecological care, self-help teaching, and sex therapy groups. The women at Aradia are currently researching for ways to attract and serve older women.

PUBLICATIONS

"America's Best Hospitals For Women." Edwin Kiester, Jr., *Ladies Home Journal*, January 1976.

For this excellent article, the author asked a diverse group of medical professionals: "What are the best American hospitals for women and why are they the best?"

The responses of the group, whose members ranged from hospital directors to women's health activists, were varied and rarely in agreement. It did, however, come up with ten best American hospitals and a list of honorable mentions. This would be a thought-provoking article for any woman facing a hospital stay.

The Directory of Women Physicians. Published by the American Medical Association.

If you feel that you must see a woman doctor and cannot get any recommendations from friends or women's centers, ask your library to order this directory. It lists *all* the women doctors in the country, not just AMA members. The doctor's age, medical education, specialties, and type of practice are listed in coded form. AMA members are specially designated and board certification is indicated.

The directory can be ordered for $10 from

>The American Medical Association
>535 North Dearborn St.
>Chicago, Ill. 60610

The most recent edition was published in 1973 and the AMA has not announced when it will be updated.

"Estrogen Therapy: The Dangerous Road to Shangri-La." *Consumer Reports*, November 1976.

Covering much of the same ground as our own chapter on estrogen, this article advocates caution in taking and prescribing estrogen. There are good explanations of the most recent studies linking ERT and endometrial cancer. Keep your eye on *Consumer Reports*—it manages to stay abreast of the most current developments in health care.

From Woman to Woman: A Gynecologist Answers Question about You and Your Body. Lucienne Lanson, M.D. Knopf, 1975, $10.00.

This book, written in a question-and-answer format, has information on a wide range of gynecological problems. It answers questions of pregnancy, sexuality, gynecological surgery, and other areas of concern, and does so thoroughly and clearly.

HealthRight—Women's Health Forum
175 Fifth Ave.
New York, N.Y. 10010
(212) 674-3660

HealthRight is concerned with women's health education and patient advocacy. They publish many informational pamphlets, including one about menopause (updated to reflect the latest findings about estrogen) and another about breast cancer. Perhaps they are best known for their publication, *HealthRight*, an excellent quarterly about women and health. The women at HealthRight would be happy to work with someone who wanted to organize a menopause group because they have received many inquiries.

The 1976 Handbook of Prescription Drugs. Richard Burack, M.D., F.A.C.P., with Fred J. Fox, M.D. Ballantine, 1976. $1.95

This book is simply excellent. In the best manner of an investigative reporter, Dr. Burack eloquently describes the failures of the pharmaceutical industry. He then supplies the consumer with the weapons to fight back: listings of brand and generic names for the most commonly prescribed drugs, price lists, and the names and addresses of suppliers of generic drugs.

Our Bodies, Ourselves. The Boston Women's Health Book Collective. Simon & Schuster, 1976. $4.95.

One of the most important works to come out of the women's movement, this is a landmark in helping women to understand their bodies. Be sure to get the new 1976 edition, completely revised and expanded, which contains an excellent section on menopause. (The women who wrote this section have taken a stronger anti-estrogen position than our chapter does.) Some sections of the book, that may be especially relevant to older women, are the sexuality section, particularly the annotated bibliography, and the sections on exercise, hysterectomy, and cancer. Although it was written by a group of young feminists, this book is informative and stimulating for women of all ages.

Talk Back to Your Doctor. Dr. Arthur Levin. Doubleday, 1975. $7.95.

This is a clear, intelligent, readable guide for consumers on how to evaluate the health and medical care they are receiving, how to get the right specialist for a problem, and how to make sure that he or she is doing the best possible job. Dr. Levin explains how to choose a doctor, what to expect from a visit, what to know about the diagnostic process, which diagnostic tests are necessary, and when to get a second opinion. He also discusses the problems of hospital and posthospital care, surgeons and surgery, and the special medical needs of women.

PHYSICAL WELL-BEING

Exercise and Diet

Aches and Pains. Robert Bristow. Pantheon Books, 1976. $8.95.

This book consists of simple exercises for "the older person" (forty and older) to alleviate the normal aches and pains of growing old or those associated with past injury, and to prevent further deterioration. It also offers techniques of massage and heat therapy. The book is conveniently organized by parts of the body and fully illustrated with photographs and drawings.

The Psychology of Successful Weight Control. Mary Catherine Tyson, M.D., and Robert Tyson, Ph.D. Nelson-Hall, 1974. $7.95.

This is a good general guide to losing weight. Success in dieting, according to the authors, is dependent upon your recognition that losing weight is an emotional matter, not just a caloric problem. The book includes diets, calorie tables, and a table of the nutritive values of foods.

Royal Canadian Air Force Exercise Plans for Physical Fitness. Pocket Books, 1972. $1.75.

These exercises are practical because they are presented in progressive order of difficulty, goals are determined by age, and the exercises take only twelve minutes to perform.

Dr. Tyson has recommended the following exercise books as especially good for keeping your whole body healthy.

Lilias N. Folan. *Lilias, Yoga & You.* Bantam, 1976. $1.75.
This book contains recommendations for other books about yoga.

Nicholas Kounovsky. *The Joy of Feeling Fit.* Avon, 1974. $3.95.

Hans Kraus. *Backaches, Stress, and Tension.* Pocket Books, 1969. $1.50.

Donald Miller. *Body-Mind: The Whole Person Health Book.* Prentice-Hall, 1974. $4.50.

Laurence E. Morehouse and Leonard Gross. *Total Fitness in 30 Minutes a Week.* Simon & Schuster, 1976. $1.95.

Bonnie Prudden. *How To Keep Slender and Fit after 30.* Pocket Books, 1972. $1.75.

Jennifer Yoels. *Re-Shape Your Body, Re-Vitalize Your Life.* Prentice-Hall, 1972. $7.95.

Beauty Care

"How You Can Look Great and Feel Sensational from Forty On." *Harper's Bazaar*, November 1974.

This is the second issue that *Harper's Bazaar* devoted to older women. There is some very good material in it—for example, an excellent article entitled "What Every Woman Should Know about Her Husband's Estate," and some sensible dos and don'ts about makeup for older women.

The Medically Based No-Nonsense Beauty Book. Deborah Chase. Knopf, 1974. $10.95.

Deborah Chase wrote this book on the assumption that women are intelligent enough to understand the scientific and medical facts of beauty care. Clearly presented, with excellent simple drawings, the text is divided into three sections—skin, eyes, and hair—with a glossary of cosmetic ingredients and terminology, and a bibliography. Brand names of the kinds of beauty products recommended are mentioned.

There is much in this book for middle-aged women. Ms. Chase explains how to care for gray hair, how estrogen creams work, why *not* to do facial exercises, and what to do about hirsutism. This book is a welcome relief from the usual pap that passes as beauty information in so many women's magazines.

Superskin—The Doctor's Guide to a Beautiful, Healthy Complexion. Jonathan Zizmor, M.D., and John Foreman. Thomas Y. Crowell Co., 1976. $7.95.

This book contains a great deal of helpful information about skin care, including the brand names for the many types of products the author recommends, and it has a fair amount of material that would interest older women, i.e., a great moisturizer for fifty cents. Our only reservations in recommending this book are that Dr. Zizmor endorses dermabrasion and chemabrasion (to which many doctors are opposed) for some women with wrinkly skin, and he does not comment on face-lifts and cosmetic surgery in general.

CANCER AND SURGERY

"After Mastectomy: Finding the Right Prosthesis." *Consumer Reports,* November 1975.

Instead of trying to rate prostheses on an excellent-to-poor scale, as they would a toaster or a lawn mower, *Consumer Reports* asked former mastectomy patients to answer questionnaires about their personal experiences in buying and wearing prostheses and over 800 women responded. *Consumer Reports* computed the satisfaction levels of various brands and put most of the forms through aging tests.

Breast Cancer: A Personal History and Investigative Report. Rose Kushner. Harcourt Brace Jovanovich, 1975. $10.00.

This is probably the best, most comprehensive book written about breast cancer, covering every aspect of the subject: history, causation, diagnosis, treatment, and rehabilitation. Rose Kushner had a mastectomy, and her book is filled with personal observations as well as valuable information. The author makes many important points: why women should be operated on by a cancer specialist and at a cancer hospital, such as Roswell Park or Sloan-Kettering, and why mastectomy and biopsy should be separated into a two step procedure.

Diary of a Pigeon Watcher. Doris Schwerin. William Morrow, 1976. $8.95.

Probing the life, forward and backward, of a woman recovering from a mastectomy, this impressionistic memoir centers around pigeon watching. The author's intense interest in a family of pigeons nesting on her windowsill gives her an understanding of both love and brutality in the natural world. This book is a reminiscence of a painful childhood, the examination of the meaning of death, and the ruminations of a middle-aged woman. Much of Ms. Schwerin's writing is rooted in pain but her tone is gentle and intelligent.

First, You Cry. Betty Rollin. J. B. Lippincott, 1976. $7.95.

Betty Rollin had a mastectomy that turned her life upside down. She writes about her anger, squeamishness, and fear with remarkable candor.

"The Greening of the Womb." Deborah Larned. *The Woman's Almanac.* Lippincott. 1976. $5.95.

This article provides a good, hard look at the controversial questions surrounding hysterectomies. Some doctors might feel that Ms. Larned is too tough on American surgeons, but she substantiates her claims with quotes from many eminent gynecologists and surgeons. Her conclusion: More and more hysterectomies are being performed every day and not all of them are necessary.

Post-Mastectomy: A Personal Guide to Physical and Emotional Recovery. Win Ann Winkler. Hawthorn, 1976. $7.95.

Although Ms. Winkler does not delve into the medical aspects of breast cancer, she does an excellent job of providing practical advice for life after breast surgery. She discusses problem areas for the woman recovering from mastectomy: sex, exercise, anxiety, and shopping for clothes, to name a few. A very useful book.

"Rush to Surgery." Joann Rodgers. *The New York Times Magazine*, September 21, 1975.

Hysterectomy is the second most frequently performed operation. In this very well-written article, Joann Rodgers asks; Should it be so frequent? Her data and her conclusions are similar to those of Deborah Larned in "The Greening of the Womb."

"What Women Don't Know about Breast Cancer." *Consumer Reports*, March 1974.

This is a short, informative article, written in a no-nonsense style, which dispels some common myths about what causes breast cancer. Included is an illustrated explanation of how to do a breast self-examination and definitions of the five types of breast cancer operations.

At the end of the article is the following list of the twenty-seven breast cancer detection centers, run by The National Cancer Institute and The American Cancer Society, where women over thirty-five years old can receive a free clinical breast examination, a mammogram, and a thermogram.

EAST

Guttman Institute
200 Madison Avenue
New York, N.Y. 10016
212-689-9797

College of Medicine and Dentistry of
    New Jersey
100 Bergen Street
Newark, N.J. 07103
201-643-6431

University of Pittsburgh School of
    Medicine
3550 Terrace Street
Pittsburgh, Pa. 15213
412-683-1620 ext. 461

Temple University—Albert Einstein
    Medical Center
York & Taber Roads
Philadelphia, Pa. 19141
215-455-8400

Wilmington Medical Center
P.O. Box 1668
Wilmington, Del. 19899
302-428-2567

Rhode Island Hospital
Rhode Island Department of Health
Davis Street
Providence, R.I. 02908
401-277-5531

SOUTH

University of Louisville School of Medicine
627 S. Floyd Street
Louisville, Ky. 40402
502-582-2111 ext. 510

St. Vincent's Medical Center
Barrs Street & St. Johns Avenue
Jacksonville, Fla. 32204
904-389-7751 ext. 8332

Vanderbilt University School of Medicine
1161 21st Avenue, South
Nashville, Tenn. 37322
615-322-7311

Emory University—Georgia Baptist Hospital
Atlanta, Ga. 30322
404-377-2472 ext. 303

Georgetown University Medical School
37th & O Streets, N.W.
Washington, D.C. 20007
202-625-7125

Duke University Medical Center
Durham, N.C. 27710
919-684-4019

MIDWEST

University of Kansas Medical Center
Rainbow Blvd. at 39th Street
Kansas City, Kans. 66103
913-831-6101

Medical College of Wisconsin
8700 W. Wisconsin Avenue
Milwaukee, Wis. 53233
414-258-2080

University of Cincinnati Medical Center
Eden & Bethesda Avenue
Cincinnati, Ohio 45229
513-872-4396

Iowa Lutheran Hospital
716 Parnell Avenue
Des Moines, Iowa 50316
515-283-5205

University of Michigan Medical Center
1414 East Ann Street
Ann Arbor, Mich. 48104
313-764-1252

Ellis Fischel State Cancer Hospital
Business Loop 70th & Garth Avenue
Columbia, Mo. 65201
314-443-3103 ext. 266 or 260

WEST

University of Oklahoma Health Sciences Center
P.O. Box 26901
Oklahoma City, Okla. 73190
405-271-5134

Mountain States Tumor Institute
151 East Bannock
Boise, Idaho 83702
208-345-1780

222 | RESOURCE DIRECTORY

WEST (Continued)

Virginia Mason Research Center
911 Seneca Street
Seattle, Wash. 98101
206-623-3700

Pacific Health Research Institute, Inc.
Alexander Young Building, Suite 542
Hotel & Bishop Streets
Honolulu, Hawaii 96813
808-531-8614

Samuel Merritt Hospital
Hawthorne & Webster Streets
Oakland, Calif. 94609
415-451-8683

University of Southern California
University Park
Los Angeles, Calif. 90007
213-225-3115 ext. 1677

University of Arizona
Arizona Medical Center
Tucson, Ariz. 35732
602-882-7401

Good Samaritan Hospital & Medical
    Center
1015 N.W. Twenty-Second Avenue
Portland, Ore. 97201
503-228-6509

St. Joseph's Hospital
1919 LaBranch
Houston, Tex. 77002
713-225-3131 ext. 269

EMOTIONAL WELL-BEING

"The Middle Years: Coping and Looking Ahead." A course taught by
    Pearl Knie, counselor and older women's advocate.

Focusing on middle-aged women, this course tries to help its students defend and redefine their value systems while they work to develop personal goals. Ms. Knie, a Gestalt-trained therapist, feels that a woman's middle years are almost as tumultuous as those of her adolescence. Ms. Knie has taught this course at the New School for Social Research in New York City and at the Women's Center of the YWCA there. To find out where the course will be held or to request information about organizing a similar course, write to:

> Pearl Knie
> 49 West 12th St.
> New York, N.Y. 10011

A Complete Guide to Therapy: From Psychoanalysis to Behavior Modification. Joel Kovel. Pantheon, 1976. $10.00.

Although this book is not easy reading, it is extremely informative and well written. *A Complete Guide To Therapy* is more than a guide. It is based on well-considered definitions of therapy. neurosis, and transference as they relate to all aspects of life. The author discusses sex therapy and points out the patient's possible gains and losses.

Dr. Kovel is a psychiatrist but he does not proselytize. This book can give you a good idea of how professional therapy might be able to help you.

Notes of a Feminist Therapist. Elizabeth Friar Williams. Praeger, 1976. $7.95.

Elizabeth Friar Williams, a feminist therapist, has put together a somewhat glib, loosely organized compendium of anecdotes, case histories, and psychological theory, which might be helpful to women who are considering therapy or those who are dissatisfied with their present therapy. Unlike some feminist therapists, she does not believe that *all* of a woman's problems are related to socialization and a sexist society. The first and perhaps the best chapter in the book, "What Is a Feminist Therapist," could easily be retitled "What Is a Good Therapist."

Shrinks, etc.: A Consumer's Guide to Psychotherapies. Thomas Kiernan. Dell, 1975. $1.95.

Thomas Kiernan tried to write a critical and comprehensive guide to psychotherapies, and, except for the first chapter, which describes gratuitously five tragic case histories, he has succeeded. The book catalogues many of the similarities and differences among the numerous psychotherapies in use today. Unfortunately, the author does not admit his own preference for behaviorism until the final chapter.

Shrinks, etc. is a helpful book for the layperson who wants to know more about therapy. Its style is clear, but uninspired.

WOMEN ALONE

Fortunately for women who live alone, many support groups have come into existence in the past few years. These groups help widows, divorcées, and single women, and have been organized by a number of institutions: churches, women's centers, and YWCAs. Some groups are more informal and are held in women's homes.

It would be very difficult to list the many organizations in this vast support system. One innovative group is described below.

>OWLA
>c/o Sylvia Borobinsky, president
>94 Claremont Ave.
>Maplewood, N.J.

Organization of Women for Legal Awareness (OWLA) primarily aids women who are in the process of being separated or divorced. The group helps women learn how to deal with lawyers and how to recognize fair treatment in their divorce proceedings. Because OWLA provides emotional help as well as legal advice, it considers itself to be the first organization of its kind in the country. Right now, in addition to its monthly meetings, it offers study sessions, educational seminars, and a newsletter. Write for more information.

Widow. Lynn Caine. Bantam, 1975. $1.75.

Everyone who has written about this book has used the word *moving*—and it is, terribly moving. *Widow* is both an account of one woman's widowhood and a guide to those in mourning. Lynn Caine is best when she recounts her feelings and the effect her husband's death had on her and their children.

Women in Transition—A Feminist Handbook on Separation and Divorce. Women in Transition, Inc. Charles Scribner's Sons, 1975. $6.95.

This excellent book began life as a pamphlet compiled by Women in Transition, Inc., a group of women from the Philadelphia Women's Center and eventually grew into the present 538-page handbook. *Women in Transition* is special because it blends hard information with sympathy in a style that is clear and direct. Divorce is not glorified as an opportunity for growth, but is treated as a painful experience.

SEXUALITY

For Yourself: The Fulfillment of Female Sexuality. Lonnie Garfield Barbach. Anchor Press, Doubleday, 1976. $3.95.

The tone of this book is straightforward and tolerant. Its purpose is to describe and to teach a treatment program that Dr. Barbach developed for women who have never experienced orgasm. There is a wealth of information here, including what kind of vibrator to buy.

Guide to Sex Therapists. Published by the American Association of Sex Educators and Counselors and Therapists.

There are thousands of unqualified sex counselors throughout the country and sex advice dispensed by people who are not competent can create a great deal of damage. In order to help people select a qualified sex therapist, the AASECT has published a state-by-state list of more than 1,150 people in the United States and abroad who have been certified by the strict standards of the association.

The guide can be ordered for $3 from

>The American Association of Sex Educators
>and Counselors and Therapists
>5010 Wisconsin Ave., N.W.
>Suite #304
>Washington, D.C. 20016

The Hite Report: A Nationwide Study of Female Sexuality. Shere Hite. Dell, 1976. $2.75.

The Hite Report has been called the most important book on the subject of female sexuality since the publication of the Masters and Johnson findings. The book contains statements from 3,019 women who answered a questionnaire of sixty questions. The result is a gargantuan source of information about women's reactions and responses to sex and sexuality.

Although the methods used were sometimes unscientific—four different questionnaires, unclear tables, overedited quotes—the overall contribution the book has made is immeasurable. It has provided a forum for women to define their own sexuality. For older women, there is a short chapter that will alleviate fears that growing old is the end of sexuality.

The Illustrated Manual of Sex Therapy. Helen Kaplan, M.D. Quadrangle, 1975. $14.95.

This is a do-it-yourself book with particularly lovely yet explicit drawings. If you are not inclined to go to a sex therapist, you can learn many of the techniques that have helped people to enjoy sex more fully.

LESBIANS

There seem to be very few resources for older women who are lesbians or who are thinking of becoming lesbians. Below is a brief list of books and articles that might serve as a starting point for women who want to know more about the lesbian experience.

226 | RESOURCE DIRECTORY

"Aging." Riki. *After You're Out: Personal Experiences of Gay Men and Lesbian Women*, edited by Karla Jay and Allen Young. Links, 1975. $4.95.

This short essay outlines the problems of being an older woman and a lesbian in our society.

Gaia's Guide 1977: For Gay Women.

A tiny book with over 2,000 listings of every kind of service and organization available, *Gaia's Guide* reveals the strength and depth of the lesbian movement.
　Send $5.00 to

        Gaia's Guide
        115 New Montgomery St.
        San Francisco, Calif. 94105
        (discreet mail order only)

"In America They Call Us Dykes." *Our Bodies, Ourselves*. The Boston Women's Health Book Collective. Simon & Schuster, 1976. $4.95.

This is a moving essay by a gay collective about the many aspects of the lesbian experience: e.g. coming out of the closet, dealing with families, and lesbian mothers.

Lesbian Women. Del Martin and Phyllis Lyon. Bantam, 1972. $1.50.

An excellent book for a woman who is thinking about lesbianism or for a woman who just wants to know more about homosexuality. It describes the growth of the lesbian movement in the United States and discusses many varieties of lesbian experiences.

"Notes of a Radical Lesbian." Martha Shelly. *Sisterhood Is Powerful*, edited by Robin Morgan. Vintage, 1970. $2.95.

The angry attitudes toward men in this essay are predictable, but it raises some points which may change your feelings about lesbianism.

One unusual organization related to the gay movement is Parents of Gays, a support group formed to help the parents of homosexuals. It publishes a booklet with a reading list and suggestions on how to deal with this situation. Send $.35 to

>Lambda Rising
>1724 20th St., N.W.
>Washington, D.C. 20009

EDUCATIONAL RESOURCES

Directories

If you would like to go back to school but for some reason cannot leave home, why not consider home study? The National Home Study Council publishes a free directory, which lists 109 accredited home study schools in the United States. In this directory are more than 200 listings ranging from accounting to dog grooming.

Write for

>The Directory of Accredited Home Study Schools
>1601 18th St., N.W.
>Washington, D.C. 20036
>(202) 659-3130

College by Mail. Jo Jensen. Arco, 1972. $4.00.

The number of college courses you can take at home is amazing—4,100 of them and all are accredited by the National University Extension Association, which is an association of sixty-four well-known colleges and universities that offer correspondence courses. *College by Mail* lists only the correspondence schools that are NUEA members. If you haven't finished high school, you can find 2,100 courses in this book, not to mention grammar school courses, graduate level courses, and certificate programs.

"Continuing Education Programs and Services for Women." Women's Bureau, U.S. Department of Labor, Washington, D.C. 20210.

This publication is described as a pamphlet, but it is really a book, and an excellent one, for any woman who wants to return to school. It is current up to 1971 and there is a 1974 supplement entitled "Continuing Education for Women: Current Developments." There are over 500 individual listings of continuing education programs for adult women and an appendix that describes related services or programs for older women. Individual copies are free; there is a charge for bulk orders.

Getting Skilled—A Guide to Trade and Technical Schools. Tom Herbert and John Coyne. Dutton, 1976. $4.95.

If you think you'd like to study auctioneering, cake decorating, horseshoeing, sign painting, violin making, or even chick sexing, you might want to consult this book. *Getting Skilled* lists all the schools that are accredited by the National Association of Trade and Technical Schools and a sampling of schools that are not accredited. This guide tells you what to look for in a trade or technical school and how to avoid unreliable ones.

The New York Times Guide to Continuing Education in America. Frances Coombs Thomson, ed. Prepared by the College Entrance Examination Board. Quadrangle Books, 1972. $4.95.

This is the most complete and comprehensive guide to education for adults. The individual schools are listed by state and the descriptions of the schools and their programs are clearly written—no codes. The entries fall into eight types of schools: universities, colleges, community colleges, junior colleges, hospitals, technical schools, vocational schools, and trade schools.

Besides its thousands of entries, the guide has a glossary, an annotated bibliography of interest to adult students, and a comprehensible explanation of how accreditation works.

Fellowships

The Clairol Loving Care Scholarship Program
c/o Business and Professional Women's Foundation
2012 Massachusetts Ave. N.W.
Washington, D.C. 20036

Clairol offers scholarships to women over thirty. If you want to go to vocational school, to two or four years of college, or to graduate school, write for an application.

Their pamphlet, "Educational Financial Aid Sources for Women," lists the limited number of scholarships that are available for women only. Some are restricted to graduate study or to specific fields. Note: The Carnegie-Mellon Mid-Career Women's Fellowship is no longer being awarded.

Write to:

> Ellen Anderson
> Clairol Loving Care Scholarship Program
> 345 Park Ave., 5th floor
> New York, N.Y. 10022

The Diuguid Fellowships

These educational fellowships are designed for women whose career and professional goals have been deferred because of marriage or for other reasons. Stipends range from $3,000 to $6,000, depending on the needs of the recipient. The qualifications for an applicant are: must be at least twenty-one years of age and have had an interruption in her career, must demonstrate financial need, and must be a resident of the southern region of the United States. For further information, write to:

> S. M. Nabritt
> 795 Peachtree St., N.E.
> Suite #484
> Atlanta, Ga. 30308

EMPLOYMENT RESOURCES

Career Centers for Women

The following private career centers represent something new—five years ago few of them existed. This is a sampling of some of the best known. Many of them have special access to jobs because they also provide affirmative-action counseling to corporations. Most of these centers are clustered on the East and West coasts. If you live somewhere in between, the best places to get vocational guidance are women's centers, YWCAs, and local colleges and universities. Some traditional employment agencies also are now beginning to focus on the particular problems of women.

Advocates for Women
256 Sutter St., 6th floor
San Francisco, Calif. 94108
(415) 391-4870

This is one of the most well-known employment centers for women. Advocates for Women calls itself a women's economic development center, which handles job openings at every level. Workshops are held and women of every background and type of experience are counseled and advised.

Career Planning Center
1623 S. LaCienega
Los Angeles, Calif.   90035
(213) 273-6633

Career Planning Center describes itself as a community-service, nonprofit organization. It offers seminars on reentering the working world, information on sex and age discrimination, vocational counseling, and a job board. Most of the services are free or there is a small fee.

Career Services for Women
382 Main St.
Port Washington, N.Y.   11050

It's encouraging to find an employment center that states that it puts special emphasis on nontraditional careers for women and on flexible employment patterns. Career Services for Women offers career workshops that would be beneficial for women returning to work, individual consultations on the Long Island job market, direct resumé referrals to employers, and a career information library. It also works with employers in developing programs to create positions that lend themselves to flexible scheduling.

Catalyst
14 E. 60th St.
New York, N.Y.   10022

Catalyst describes itself as a national nonprofit organization that helps to expand career opportunities for college-educated women. It has an excellent reputation for helping women, and the services it offers are almost too numerous to mention. One outstanding free publication is Catalyst's "National Network of Local Resource Centers." This eight-page, state-by-state listing includes information about many programs of continuing education and career-planning centers. Especially helpful to older women is Catalyst's "Education Opportunities Series." These ten booklets, covering fields ranging from business administration to urban planning, are designed to help returning students identify and evaluate an appropriate educational program.

Center for Displaced Homemakers
2435 Maryland Ave.
Baltimore, Md. 21218
(301) 243-5000

Although it serves the same type of woman as its sister agency in California (see below), the Baltimore Center for Displaced Homemakers is a bit different. This one-month-old agency wants to develop a full job placement program serving both employers and displaced homemakers. Right now, the center provides counseling, workshops, and referrals for job training. Soon it hopes to develop a program that would help women create their own jobs, such as small home industries and small businesses.

All of the women who work at the Center for Displaced Homemakers were at one time displaced homemakers themselves and they represent a combination of paid workers and volunteers.

Civic Center and Clearing House, Inc.
14 Beacon St.
Boston, Mass. 02108
(617) 227-1762

Fifteen years ago Civic Center and Clearing House was founded as a non-profit agency to offer counseling and placement to volunteers. Today it still performs that function but also provides a Career and Vocational Advisory Service (CVAS) with counseling, information on continuing education, referrals, internships, and apprenticeships. CVAS is a member of the Women's Work Cooperative, a coalition of ten agencies, which share job listings.

"Project Re-Entry," a combination of job counseling and an on-the-job training program for women over thirty-five, is a new, exciting program sponsored by the Civic Center and Clearing House. Designed to provide an introduction (or reintroduction) to the working world, Project Re-Entry consists of six weeks of job counseling and then placement in the unsalaried internship or apprenticeship of a woman's choice.

Fees for all Civic Center and Clearing House services are moderate.

Displaced Homemaker's Center
Mills College
P.O. Box #9996
Oakland, Calif. 94613
(415) 632-4600

This agency was the first of its kind in the country. It serves women who are over thirty-five years old, have worked as homemakers most of their adult lives, and have lost the emotional and financial support of their husbands—in other words, women who have nowhere else to turn.

This is not a job placement agency; it is a job creation program, which goes right to the heart of the problem. Displaced Homemaker's Center finds an area in the community that needs a service, develops a job to fill that need, then obtains funding to finance the new position. Finally, a displaced homemaker is hired to fill the job.

Displaced Homemaker's Center also creates and subsidizes internships to provide training for women as well as offering its own workshops. Another service is the arrangement of a volunteer contract, whereby a woman works as a professional volunteer in order to gain needed experience.

EVE Women's Center
Kean College of New Jersey
Union, N.J. 07083

EVE stands for education, vocation, and employment. This women's center offers a range of services: educational and vocational counseling, vocational interest testing, resumé consultation, workshops and group discussions, a library, and resource files. EVE's fees are moderate and there is no charge for an introductory interview. It offers a program, called EPIC, for older women who wish to enter or reenter college. EPIC is designed to ease their reentry into the classroom and to provide alternative ways to earn a degree.

Federation Employment and Guidance Service (FEGS)
215 Park Avenue South
New York, N.Y. 10003

This organization is a nonprofit and nonsectarian vocational service operated by the Federation of Jewish Philanthropies of New York. It offers a wide range of services including educational and vocational guidance, skills training, and psychological testing, in addition to the job placement services. Some of the job counselors are especially concerned with the problems of older women returning to the labor force. In addition to its New York City facilities, FEGS has outreach programs on Long Island and in Westchester.

Flexible Careers
Room 703
37 South Wabash Ave.
Chicago, Ill. 60603

Flexible Careers is a nonprofit career consultation service that focuses on the employment and career needs of Chicago area women of all ages, backgrounds, and skills. Its counselors feel they are experts at helping the woman who doesn't fit into easily defined job categories. They help with resumé preparation, development of job campaigns, and direct job leads.

Higher Education Resource Services
Box 1901
Providence, R.I.   02912
(401) 863-2197

If you are interested in starting to teach at the university level or perhaps in resuming a teaching career you began many years ago, this multiservice center would be worth investigating.

Project Hers

This group was organized early in 1972 to help create a national network of professional women, which would foster the progress of women just entering the academic profession. Services available are: a talent bank, search, referral, and placement services, follow-ups on all referrals, and an Academic Career Information Service. HERS has a branch in Philadelphia. Its address is:

> HERS-Midatlantic
> Fourth Floor, 4025 Chestnut St.
> University of Pennsylvania
> Philadelphia, Pa. 19104

Janice LaRouche Associates
333 Central Park West
New York, N.Y.   10025
(212) 663-0970

Janice LaRouche has an excellent reputation for helping women with all kinds of work-related problems. Ms. LaRouche and her associate, Penelope Russianoff, hold courses at the New School and at a midtown YWCA. They offer four basic programs: career planning, career advancement, assertiveness training, and "Becoming Your Independent Self." The career planning workshop would be the most beneficial for women who are thinking about returning to work

Options for Women, Inc.
8419 Germantown Ave.
Philadelphia, Pa. 19118
(215) CH 2-4955

Options for Women describes itself as one of the most comprehensive organizations in the country serving the needs of women. It has group and individual vocational and educational counseling and testing, and job placement at all levels. This agency is an independent nonprofit corporation whose fees are described as moderate.

Washington Opportunities for Women (WOW)
1649 K St., N.W.
Washington, D.C. 20006
(202) 638-4868

The WOW career center is a career-planning, job-counseling, and referral organization serving women and employers in the Washington metropolitan area. WOW was established seven years ago as an experimental effort by a few dedicated women who were looking for answers to their work-related problems and found there was no place to go. During the last year alone, WOW has served 10,000 women from all segments of the Washington area. WOW has six branches along the Eastern Seaboard:

>   Atlanta Wider Opportunities for Women
>   161 Peachtree St., N.E.
>   Room #310
>   Atlanta, Ga. 30303
>   (404) 656-5923
>
>   Baltimore New Directions for Women
>   1123 North Eutaw St.
>   Baltimore, Md. 21201
>   (301) 383-5579
>
>   Wider Opportunities for Women, Boston
>   C.F. Hurley Building
>   Government Center
>   Cambridge and Staniford Sts.
>   Boston, Mass. 02114
>   (617) 727-8978

Opportunities for Women
72 Pine St.
Providence, R.I. 02903
(401) 421-1410

Richmond Women on the Way
308 Cary Street
Richmond, Va. 23219
(804) 770-6001

WISE-WOW
5 North Main St.
White River Junction, Vt. 05001
(802) 295-3136

Women's Educational and Industrial Union
356 Boylston St.
Boston, Mass. 02116
(617) 536-5651

The Women's Educational and Industrial Union is a nonprofit social service organization, founded in 1877. Among its many services, Career Services would be the one most helpful to older women. In addition to providing counseling, job placement, and a resource room, Career Services holds "Career Clinics for Returners" on a regular basis. Counseling and use of the resource room are free and fees for other services vary.

The Women's Opportunities Center
148 Administration Building
University of California Extension
Irvine, Calif. 92664

This center is exclusively for women who want to change their lives after an interruption of education and/or career. Staffed almost entirely by volunteers, the center was opened in September 1970. Through the center many women are directed to further their education. Others, who are ready to enter the job market, are advised on techniques of job finding. A membership fee of $10 entitles you to counseling, the newsletter, the use of the library, and reduced fees for workshops and groups.

Publications

"Careers for Women in the 70's." Women's Bureau, U.S. Department of Labor, Washington, D. C. 20210.

Stuffed with figures and percentages, this clearly written booklet can shed some light on your career choice—what percentage of workers in what fields are women and how many job openings there are annually.

"Part-Time Work: When Less Is More." Carol Greenwald. *Ms.* May 1976.

This is an excellent article by a woman who held a part-time position as assistant vice-president and economist, Federal Reserve Bank of Boston. Although Ms. Greenwald's desire to work part time was predicated by the needs of a small child, the information she provides is valuable to any woman.

Ms. Greenwald deftly works her way through the standard arguments against serious part-time work: not enough time on the job and the problems with state taxes and health insurance. Her calculations may help you determine if your employer could divide your job into two part-time jobs. This idea might sound quite revolutionary, but the author makes it seem both practical and workable.

"Volunteerism—What It's All About." Berkeley: Women and Volunteerism Task Force, 1973. $1.50 from NOW Headquarters, 423 13th St., Suite #1001, Washington, D.C. 20004.

NOW's position on volunteering is radical and right on target in many instances. It makes the distinction between service-oriented volunteering and change-oriented volunteering. If you are or ever will be a volunteer, this pamphlet merits your consideration.

Women, Work and Volunteering. Herta Loeser. Beacon, 1974. $4.75.
(This book can be ordered for $4.95 ppd. from The Civic Center and Clearing House, Inc., 14 Beacon St., Boston, Mass. 02108.)

This book is a must for any woman who does or would like to do volunteer work, or who is thinking of returning to work but has cold feet. Herta Loeser is not writing about the traditional approach to volunteering—she believes volunteering can train you for a career, add to the satisfaction of your ordinary working day, and help you to affect social change. She is a feminist and offers cogent arguments in support of volunteering. The chapter "Feminism and Volunteering" should be read in conjunction with NOW's position (see above).

This book contains many excellent resources, including a chapter on "How to Locate a Suitable Volunteer Job" and a thorough description of the many different categories of volunteer work. The highly informative commentary, based on years of experience, is sprinkled with case histories of successful volunteers.

What Color Is Your Parachute? Richard Nelson Bolles. Ten Speed Press, 1972. Box 4310, Berkeley, Calif. 94704. $4.95 plus $.25 for postage and handling.

This book is jam-packed with addresses, footnotes, book descriptions, and a plethora of useful tips and suggestions. Mr. Bolles describes it as a "practical manual for job-hunters and career changers." His evaluations of our "Neanderthal" job-hunting system are almost scary, but his ways of beating it are terribly simple and sensible.

Women's Work. A bimonthly career magazine for women.

The only magazine of its kind in the country, *Women's Work* tells how to get jobs, change careers, keep jobs, how to start a business, how to dress for work, how to create jobs for yourself, and much more. The price is $4 for six issues. Write to:

>Women's Work
>1649 K St., N.W.
>Washington, D.C. 20006

Women's Work Book. Karin Aberbanel and Gonnie McClung Siegel. Praeger, 1975. $4.95.

There is a great deal of practical information in this book, which would be useful to any woman looking for a job, regardless of her background and experience. Some of the tips offered by the authors are: How to deal with a sexist interviewer, how to decode job advertisemnts, and how to tap the hidden job market. There is also an enormous directory of job-finding and career-building resources. This is a good, helpful book.

238 | RESOURCE DIRECTORY

GENERAL RESOURCES

National Women's Organizations

National Organization For Women
423 13th St., suite #1001
Washington, D.C. 20004
(202) 347-2279

This is by far the largest feminist organization in the United States. Activities vary greatly among the individual chapters, and some chapters are more concerned than others with older women's problems. For example, the New York chapter has a Standing Committee on Older Women, which has sponsored many different programs, while right across the river in New Jersey, there hasn't been much happening for older women.

NOW has a national task force on older women, which is very active.

NOW's Task Force on Older Women
3800 Harrison St.
Oakland, Calif. 94611

This group, headed by Tish Sommers, has been doing wonderful things for older women. They have an excellent newsletter (four issues for $1) and a thorough bibliography on menopause. The Task Force is working on reform of the social security system and help for the displaced homemaker. Write for their list of excellent publications. A contribution would be "wildly welcomed."

YWCA
600 Lexington Ave.
New York, N.Y. 10022
(212) 753-4700

This organization has grown out of its staid old image and is running some of the most exciting women's programs in the country. Don't confuse it with the YMCA—they are separate organizations and have goals and images that are very different. In general, YWCAs are an important resource for older women.

Two excellent programs for older women are described below.

Women in Midstream
University of Washington YWCA
4224 University Way, NE
Seattle, Wash. 98105
(206) 632-4747

Women in Midstream describes itself as a study group. Some of the services it offers are a newsletter, a speakers' bureau, round tables, tape recordings, and a library. The group started as an ad hoc committee sponsored by the University YMCA, Seattle, to survey women's experiences with menopause. For two years the women in the group reviewed books, medical journals, and popular magazines, interviewed health professionals, and talked with other women. One of their conclusions was that menopause cannot be separated from other life experiences.

As a study group, WIM has been primarily concerned with organizing and disseminating information drawn from women's personal experiences with menopause. They sent questionnaires to all parts of the United States and have received about 700 responses. Right now the questionnaires are being compiled and a book is in preparation.

YWCA
West Suburban Area
1 South Park
Lombard, Ill. 60148

"Over Forty and Now What?" is a booklet prepared by the YWCA of West Suburban Area in conjunction with the Women's Law Caucus of Lewis University and the Illinois Humanities Council. The booklet, which costs $3.00 (including mailing costs), was intended to be just for local distribution, but it contains so much practical information about wills, credit ratings, social security, and so forth, that women across the nation have been using it.

"Over Forty and Now What?" is one part of the older women's program at the Lombard YWCA—there are support groups, lectures, and divorce counseling. The women there are constantly searching for new ways to help middle-aged women.

Local Women's Organizations

Women's centers can be wonderful sources of help. Of course, the quality and services vary greatly from location to location. The description of the

240 | RESOURCE DIRECTORY

Women's Resource Center, below, will give you an idea of the kinds of services you might find. To locate a women's center near you, check the list of general source books at the end of this directory or inquire at local colleges or universities.

Women's Resource Center
1406 Pine St.
Boulder, Col.   80302
(303) 447-9670

This women's center is making a concerted effort to reach out to older women. It can make doctor referrals, and it has an Older Women's Task Force, which is basically a support group. The center has held many workshops on topics that concern middle-aged women—sexuality, menopause, and reentering the job market.

READING LIST

Nonfiction

Ruth Carson. "Your Menopause," Public Affairs Pamphlet #447.

This pamphlet, directed toward middle-class women, was written in 1970, and therefore needs some updating. It has a short bibliography, however, which might be of interest to some women.
   Write to

> Public Affairs Pamphlets
> 381 Park Ave. South
> New York, N.Y. 10022

Vidal Clay. *Women: Menopause and Middle Age.* KNOW, Inc. P.O. Box 86031, Pittsburgh, Pa. 15221. 1977. $5.95.

This book, to be published after this directory goes to press, is sure to be excellent, as are all of the publications from this fine feminist press.

Alex Comfort. *A Good Age.* Crown, 1976. $9.95.

Dr. Alex Comfort, the author of *The Joy of Sex*, is an outstanding gerontologist. *A Good Age* is an absolutely stunning book, filled with lovely drawings, mezzotints, and silk-screen prints of older people, and sprinkled with epigrams about old age and sketches of famous older people. The long introduction by Dr. Comfort is followed by an alphabetized list of topics ranging from Quackery to Living in Sin. There is vigor and honesty in this book, which speaks to us of passion and intelligence, not of arthritis and resignation.

Janice Delaney, Mary Jane Lupton, and Emily Toth. *The Curse: A Cultural History of Menstruation.* Dutton, 1976. $9.95.

Even though only three chapters of this absorbing book are devoted to menopause, *The Curse* offers fresh information and insight. The authors, who are professors of English, have included a fascinating discussion of the images of menopausal women in literature, ranging from Chaucer's works to those of John O'Hara. Like *Menstruation and Menopause*, *The Curse* shows that women continue to suffer from the centuries-old menstrual taboos of primitive societies and the frightening and inaccurate view of menopause that medicine, religion, and history have provided. The authors weave this thesis through their examination of menstruation in myth, poetry, fiction, drama, and folktale.

Janet Harris. *The Prime of Ms. America: The American Woman at 40.* Signet. $1.50.

Although Janet Harris writes from a decidedly upper-middle-class perspective, her commentary on middle-aged women in our society should produce a flash of recognition from all older women. The author is obviously a strong feminist, but *The Prime of Ms. America* is sensible and sincere.

It covers a wide range of topics including sex, identity, changing relationships, and an aging body. In her treatment of these, Ms. Harris integrates her own experience, the feelings of the eighty women she interviewed, and the opinions of the authorities in each field.

Lillian Hellman. *Pentimento.* Signet, 1974. $1.95.

———. *An Unfinished Woman.* Bantam, 1974. $1.50.

These books are simply exquisite. *Pentimento* is a continuation of the recollections begun in *An Unfinished Woman.* Although the people she has known and the things she has done are fascinating, nothing is more so than Lillian Hellman herself—fiery, impetuous, ambivalent, and brilliant. Her memoirs will not tell you how to cope with middle age but they do reveal an older woman with extraordinary intelligence and insight.

A. E. Hotchner. *Doris Day: Her Own Story.* Bantam, 1975. $1.95.

Doris Day's Hollywood image as the archetypical happy-go-lucky virgin is completely false. She has had a tough time in her personal relationships and suffered financial disaster because her husband, with the help of an unscrupulous lawyer, mismanaged her life's earnings. After reading this interesting but sad book, you may feel that Doris Day contributed greatly to her own difficulties, but you will have to admire her tenacity and resiliency.

Olga Knopf, M.D. *Successful Aging: The Facts and Fallacies of Growing Old.* Viking, 1975. $8.95.

When Dr. Knopf was in her middle fifties, she became interested in the relationship between middle-aged adults and their aged parents. This curiosity led to a twenty-year study of the problems of the elderly, and to this very fine book, written for elderly people who are fairly healthy but who need reassurance that life isn't over. The author, now an active eighty-five-year-old practicing psychiatrist, has tried to increase the self-awareness of older people and to induce them to accept situations they cannot change.

Joseph Lash. *Eleanor: The Years Alone.* New American Library, 1973. $1.95.

In the seventeen years following her husband's death, Eleanor Roosevelt made her mark in politics and international diplomacy. She had an active interest in world affairs until the day of her death. This excellent book tells the story of a woman who suffered greatly in her personal relationships but who did not fail to lead a courageous and satisfying life.

Eda LeShan. *The Wonderful Crisis of Middle Age.* Warner, 1973. $1.75.

This is a sensible, comforting book, filled with miniature case histories and anecdotes about middle-aged people. Ms. LeShan's thesis is that middle age is a time to enjoy yourself and to be yourself, and one has the feeling that she herself has agonized over the problems she describes and analyzes. The one flaw in this book is Ms. LeShan's view of the relations between men and women: e.g., that men should make the major moral decisions for the family and that most liberated women of her generation have no desire to have their husbands share equally in the housework.

Golda Meir. *My Life.* Dell, 1975. $1.95.

This is an inspiring book which transcends the dimensions of a political memoir and should be read by any woman who thinks life ends at menopause. At age fifty Golda Meir was appointed Israel's first ambassador to Russia and at age sixty-seven, she retired as foreign minister of Israel, only to be called back as its prime minister. Since it is impossible for Mrs. Meir to describe her life without discussing the birth and development of Israel, her autobiography may be overly historical for some readers. For the most part, however, it is a moving reminder that women can do anything they want to do.

Zoe Moss. "It Hurts to Be Alive and Obsolete: The Aging Woman." *Sisterhood Is Powerful*, edited by Robin Morgan. Vintage. $2.95.

Zoe Moss is the pseudonym of a forty-three-year-old woman who is very angry about the prejudices against older women in our social and sexual systems. In this essay, the author points out many of the ironies concerning middle-aged women in our culture: that older black women are always considered sexual beings and that older men mature, while older women become obsolescent. Ms. Moss's accusations are just, but her tone is bitter.

Anais Nin. *The Diary of Anais Nin.* , vol. v, 1947–1955. Harcourt Brace Jovanovich, 1975. $2.95.

Anais Nin has made the diary into an art form. With vivid and lyrical descriptions and self-analyses, she explores in this volume some of the events that befall many middle-aged women, i.e., death of parents, gynecological surgery.

Gail Sheehy. *Passages: Predictable Crises of Adult Life.* Dutton, 1976. $9.95.

Passages is a descriptive analysis of the emotional stages of adult life into which Ms. Sheehy artfully weaves 115 case histories. She points out that men and women are rarely in the same psychological place at the same time with regard to work, family commitments, and sexual needs. This explains the polarization that can occur between the sexes. One flaw: She is a little too eager to apply the word *growth* to every happening in an adult's life. Despite this "positive thinking," *Passages* offers much worth considering.

Paula Weidegger. *Menstruation and Menopause: The Physiology and Psychology of the Myth and Reality.* Knopf, 1975. $10.

In this very important book, Paula Weidegger examines the historical, sociological, and psychological foundations of menstruation and menopause. She relates much of this factual material to the comments of the 558 women who responded to her questionnaire. There is an excellent chapter on menopause. Weidegger shows that in spite of a new willingness to discuss their bodies, women still regard menstruation and menopause as social embarrassments—in her words, we've simply internalized the menstrual huts of old.

Journal

Prime Time—"a feminist journal for older women or for the liberation of women in the prime of life."

Prime Time has original articles, reprints, opinions, reader's letters, and a news and views section. *Prime Time* is unique: the only existing publication for, by, and about older women. It costs $7.00 for six issues.

Write to

>Prime Time
>420 West 46th St.
>New York, N.Y. 10036

Fiction

Thanks are due to Corinne Mattuck for her suggestions. Also, see the bibliography, "Age Is Becoming," under General Sourcebooks below for more listings.

Dorothy Bryant. *Ella Price's Journal.* Lippincott, 1972.
Evan Connell. *Mrs. Bridge.* Viking, 1958.
Doris Lessing. *The Summer before the Dark.* Knopf, 1973. $7.95.
Alison Lurie. *The War between the Tates.* Warner, 1976. $1.95.
May Sarton. *Kinds of Love.* Norton, 1970 $6.95.
———. *Mrs. Stevens Hears the Mermaids Singing.* Norton, 1975. $2.45.

———. *Journal of a Solitude.* Norton, 1973. $6.95.
———. *Crucial Conversations.* Norton, 1975. $5.95.
Muriel Spark. *Momento Mori.* Avon, 1971. $1.65.
———. *The Prime of Miss Jean Brodie.* Dell, 1966. $.95.

General Sourcebooks

"Age Is Becoming." Compiled by a grant from NOW's Legal Defense and Education Fund, this selective bibliography of current literature on the impact of aging on women has solid lists of annotated fiction and biography, and there are many entries from journals and government reprints. Enthusiastically recommended.

Write and send $2.50 to:

> Interface Bibliographers
> 3018 Hillegass Avenue
> Berkeley, California 94705

The New Women's Survival Sourcebook. Knopf, 1975. $5.00.
PsychoSources. Bantam, 1973. $5.00.
The Woman's Almanac. Lippincott, 1976. $6.95.
Women in Transition (see Health Resources: Emotional Well-Being)
Women, Work, and Volunteering. (see Employment Resources).
Women's Workbook (see Employment Resources).

INDEX

Abdominal cramping, 96
Ablation, therapeutic, 111
Abnormal bleeding, 25–26
Acidosis, 152
Acne, 67, 68
"Action cure" for worry, 162
Adair, John, 136
Addison's disease, 4
Adrenal glands, 10, 52, 57
Advertising industry, 39–40
Agar, 149–150
Aging skin, 171
Alcohol, 145, 171
American Board of Obstetrics and Gynecology, 98
American Board of Plastic Surgery, 163
American Cancer Society, 82, 103
American Medical Association, 152
American Society of Plastic and Reconstructive Surgeons, 163
Androgen, 54–55, 112
 production of, 52
 side effects from, 67–68

Anorexia nervosa, 23
Anovulatory cycles, 89
Anxiety, 23, 26, 35, 36, 125, 131, 138, 142
 tension treatments, 162
Arms, surgical correction of, 168
Artificial breast, 109
Asthma, 70
Atkins, Robert C., 152
Atkins diet, 152
Atrophic (shrinking or thinning) changes, 26–29
Attractiveness, sexual, 113–114
Autosuggestion, 152
Average woman's life span (U.S.), 11, 144
Ayds diet candy, 150–151

Behavior modification, for dieting, 151–152
Belgium, 9, 13
Berman, Edgar, 3–4
Bernard, Jesse, 140–141
Bilateral oophorectomy, 95, 99

247

Bilateral salpingo-oophorectomy, 95
Birth control, 10, 24–25
Birth control pills, 51
Body configuration changes, 31–32
Body surgery, cosmetic, 168–169
Bonnadonna, Gianni, 110
Boston Women's Health Book Collective, 14
Bowel movements, 33
Breast, cosmetic surgery for, 168
Breast cancer, 82, 99–111
   biopsy, 104–105
   detection, 101
   estrogens and, 100–101
   risk factor, 99–100
   self-examination, 101–102
     how to do, 102
   surgery and, 105–111
     after care treatment, 109–110
     endocrine manipulation, 110–111
     prostheses, 109
     recovery period, 108–109
     "stage" of the cancer, 105–107
     type of, 107–108
   X-ray screening, 102–104
Breast examination (free), 220–221
Breathlessness, 13
Buttocks, surgical correction of, 168

Calcium loss, 11, 30–31
Cancer, 11, 15, 79
   breast, 82, 99–111
     biopsy, 104–105
     detection, 101
     estrogens and, 100–101
     risk factor, 99–101
     self-examination, 101–102
     surgery and, 105–111
     X-ray screening, 102–104
   of the cervix, 62, 85–88
     prognosis after treatment, 88
     treatment of, 87–88
   endometrial, 51, 60, 61, 88–90
   endometriosis and 78
   estrogen therapy and, 61–63
   hysterectomy and, 82–93
     cervical intraepithelial neoplasia, 83–85
     the cervix, 85–88
     lining of the uterus, 88–90
     ovaries, 90–93
Carbohydrate metabolism, estrogen therapy and, 60–61
Carcinoma in situ, 83, 84
Castile soap, 169
Catherine of Aragon, 139
Celibacy, choosing, 115–116
Centenarians, 144
Cerebral thrombosis, 60
Cervical intraepithelial neoplasia (CIN), 83–85, 86
   prognosis for, 85
   treatment of, 84
Cervical mucus, 55
Cervical polyps, 25
Cervicitis (inflammation of the cervix), 25
Cervix, cancer of, 62, 85–88
Cervix (mouth of the womb), 21, 27, 28, 53, 72
Change of life. See Menopause
Checkups, 33–34
Chemotherapy, 110
Childhood and Society (Erikson), 133
Children, communicating with, 47–48
China, 7, 32
Chisholm, Shirley, 4
Chronic coughing, 80
Cigarette smoking, 145, 171
Clooney, Rosemary, 37
Colposcopy, 84
Committee on National Priorities, 3

Condoms, 25
Constipation, 33
Contraception, 10, 24-25
Cosmetic surgery, 162-169
  body image and personality,
    162-163
  decision for, 163
  improving skin care and, 165-169
    altering facial features, 167
    the body, 168-169
    the breast, 168
    cryosurgery, 166-167
    dermabrasion, 167
    dermaplaning, 166
    face-lifts, 167-168
    face peels, 165-166
  reasons not to have, 165
  as a serious enterprise, 169
  what it can and cannot do,
    164-165
  when it's beneficial, 163-164
County Medical Society, 98
Crile, George, 108
Cryosurgery, 166-167
Cryotherapy, 84, 85
*Curse, The: A Cultural History of
    Menopause* (Delaney and
    Lupton), 6, 7
Cystocele (bladder descent), 28
Cystoscopy, 81, 93

Darrow, C. M., 133, 140
Delaney, Janice, 6, 7
Depressed life-style, 38
Depression, mental, 6, 8, 13, 31, 35,
    36, 41-43, 57, 114, 131, 132
  signs of, 41
Dermabrasion, 167
Dermaplaning, 166
Deutsch, Helene, 6
Devereaux, George, 7
Diaphragm, 25

Diet, 147-154
  changes in calorie needs, 146-147
  emotional factors in reducing,
    149-150
  how to choose, 149
  reducing plans, 150-154
    Atkins diet, 152
    Ayds candy, 150-151
    behavior modification, 151-152
    best for weight loss, 154
    fads and miracle methods,
      153-154
    fasting, 152-153
    group approach, 150
    Stillman diet, 152
  special problems, 147-148
  vitamin supplements, 148
  weight and, 145-146
Diet tablets, 149-150
Diethylstilbesterol (DES), 86-87
Dilatation and curettage (D & C),
    26, 74, 79, 91
Dizziness, 13, 57
Dysplasia, 83, 84

Emotions, 6-7, 8, 35-50
  and communicating with children,
    47-48
  depression, 6, 8, 13, 31, 35, 36
    41-43, 57, 114, 131, 132
  fear, 38-39
  healthy type of, 50
  help from friends, 47
  intellectual growth, 49
  meeting new men, 43-44
  menopausal mother, 45
  psychotherapy for, 45-46
  realistic expectations, 49-50
  single woman, 43, 44-45
  society and, 39-41
  stress points, 36-38
  therapists and, 46-47

Emotions (*cont.*)
   virtues of self-indulgence, 48–49
Emphysema, 145
Endocrine glands, 12
Endocrine manipulation, 110-111
Endometrial cancer, 51, 60, 61, 88–90
   cure rates for, 90
Endometrial polyps, 25
Endometriosis, 74–78
   cancer and, 78
   symptoms, 76–77
   treatment of, 77–78
Endometrium, 53, 55, 59, 62, 75, 79, 88–90
Epilepsy, 70
Erikson, Erik, 6–7, 133
Erotic movies, 124
Estradiol, 11
Estriol, 11
Estrogen, 11, 12, 15–16, 23, 24, 32, 51–71, 77, 79, 89, 95, 113, 148
   in animals, 54
   basic evaluation and, 64–71
      decision for, 66
      follow-up, 69–70
      how much to take, 66–67
      natural or synthetic compounds, 68–69
      responsible physician, 70–71
      route of administration, 69
      who should not take, 65–66
      who should take, 64–65
   breast cancer incidence, 100–101
   "female principle" and, 52
   measuring levels of, 55–56
   oral, 29, 113
   other sex hormones and, 54–55, 67–68
   production of, 10, 12, 52, 54
      at menopause, 56–57
   puberty and, 53–54
   role of, 53
   side effects and, 57–64
      cancer, 61–63
      evaluating the risks, 58–60
      inconclusive studies, 61
      medical need, 63–64
      prospective studies, 57–58
      retrospective studies, 58
      risk versus benefit ratio, 60–61
Estrogen binding test, 111
Estrogen creams, 27, 32, 69, 128
Estrone, 11
Estrus behavior, 54
Everything You Always Wanted To Know About Sex (but Were Afraid to Ask) (Reuben), 16–17
Excessive sweating, 13
Exercise, 154–159, 171
   aids for, 158–159
   choosing your own, 156
   in groups, 156
   at home, 157–158
   reason for, 155
   for relaxation, 161

Face-lifts, 167–168
Face peels, 165–166
Facial features, altering, 167
Fantasy, sexual use of, 125
Fasting, 152–153
Fatigue, 20, 57
FDA Drug Bulletin, 59
Fear, 38–39
Fibroids (leiomyomata uteri), 73–75
   diagnosing, 74–75
   intramural and submucosal, 73–74
Flabbiness, 32
Follicle stimulating hormone (FSH), 23
Food and Drug Administration (FDA), 58, 59, 70

Ford, Betty, 82
France, 9, 13
Freud, Sigmund, 6, 41–42, 135
Friedan, Betty, 4
Friendships, reviving, 48
Future of Marriage, The (Bernard), 141

Gandhi, 135
Gauguin, Eugène Paul, 131
Goya, Francesco, 135
Great Britain, 9, 13

Hair, thinning of, 169–170
Halstead Radical Mastectomy, 107–108
Headaches, 12–13, 16, 33, 57
Healthy emotions, 50
Henry VIII (king), 139
Her Infinite Variety (Hunt), 7
Holmes Stress Scale, 5
Homosexuality, 118
Hormone balance, 12
Hormones. *See* names of hormones
Hot flush (or hot flash), 12, 13, 14, 22–24, 33, 56–57, 148
Human Sexual Response (Masters and Johnson), 137–138
Humphrey, Hubert, 3, 82
Hunt, Morton, 7
Hyperplasia, 78–80
  prognosis for, 79–80
Hypertension, 60, 159–160
Hypothalamus glands, 23
Hysterectomy, 11, 16, 21, 72–98
  benign conditions and, 73–82
    endometriosis, 75–78
    fibroids, 73–75
    hyperplasia and polyps, 78–80
    pelvic relaxation, 80–82
  cancer and, 82–93
    cervical intraepithelial
    neoplasia, 83–85
    the cervix, 85–88
    lining of the uterus, 88–90
    ovaries, 90–93
  meaning of, 72–73
  preparation for, 93–94
  surgery and, 94–98
    recovery period, 96–97
    types of operations, 94–96
    unnecessary surgery, 98

Impatience, 13
Impotence, 124, 137
Incontinence, stress, 29
India, 32
Insomnia, 33, 41
Intellectual growth, 49
International Health Foundation, 9, 12–13
Intra-uterine device (IUD), 25
Intravenous pylogram (IVP), 80, 88, 93
Irritability, 13
Isometric exercises, 157
Italy, 9, 13

Johnson, Lyndon B., 4
Johnson, Virginia E., 137–138
Joint pains, 13
Jung, Carl Gustav, 135

Kegel's exercises, 29, 81
Keratoses, 171
Knauer, Emil, 52
Kraines, Ruth J., 8
K-Y jelly, 27, 113, 128

Labia, 54
Labia majora, 28
Ladies' Home Journal, The, 36
Lassitude, 13
Leaf, Alexander, 144

252 | INDEX

Lear, Martha Weinman, 135
Lesbianism, 118
Levinson, D. J., 133, 134-135, 136, 139, 140
Lewis, Sinclair, 135
Libido, change in, 33
Lincoln, Abraham, 4
Lipid metabolism, estrogen therapy and, 60-61
Liver function, estrogen therapy and, 61
Liver spots, 171
Lumpectomy, 108
Lung cancer, 145
Lupton, Mary Jane, 6, 7
Lymph glands, 106
Lymph nodes, 72, 95
Lymphadenectomy, 95

Male Climacteric, The (Ruebsaat), 131, 138
Male menopause, 130-143
   age at mid-life crisis, 139-140
   family and, 139
   manifestations, 130-131
   precipitants of, 131-136
   and relationship with women, 140-142
   sexual changes, 137-138
   sexual therapy, 142-143
   symptoms, 131
Mammography, 102-103
Marfan's syndrome, 4
Marriage, 116-121
   alternatives to, 118-121
   choosing, 116
   enriching sex life in, 116-117
Massage, 159
Massage parlors, 123
Masters, William H., 137-138
Masturbation, 112, 126-127

Mead, Margaret, 135
Menarche, the, 36, 54
Menopause:
   diagnosis of, 18
   emotions and, 6-7, 35-50
   estrogen treatment, 51-71
   and hysterectomy, 72-98
   increase in sexual drive after, 17
   as an individual experience, 15
   male, 130-143
   meaning of, 3-17
   reading list, 240-245
   physiology of, 9-16
   publications, 214-220, 222, 229, 236-237
   resource directory, 201-245
   sex at, 122-129
   stress and, 5-6, 36-38
   symptoms and changes, 18-34
   women on, 7-9
      interviews with, 172-200
      women's organizations, 238-240
Menopause, The: A Study of the Attitudes of Women in Belgium, France, Great Britain, Italy and West Germany (International Health Foundation), 13
Menstruation and Menopause: The Physiology and Psychology, the Myth and the Reality (Weideger), 7
Methyl cellulose, 149-150
Middle Age and Aging (Neugarten, ed.), 136
Milk, 53
"Mini-menopause," 112
Mink, Patsy, 3-4
Mohave Indians, 7
Moore, Charles, 107

Mucosa (lining) of the vagina, 27
Muscle pains, 13
Myocardial infarction, 60

National Academy of Science, 152
National Center for Health Statistics, 61
National Institute of Health, 152
Needle aspiration, 104
Nervousness, 13
Neugarten, Bernice L., 8, 136, 139, 140
Newsweek, 61
Nitrogen balance, metabolic changes in, 60

Obesity, 32
Obstetric and Gynecology Advisory Committee (Food and Drug Administration), 59
O'Neill, Eugene, 135
Oophorectomy, 21, 101
Oral estrogen, 29, 113
Oral sex, 124
Osteoporosis, 11, 30-31, 67, 148
Our Bodies, Ourselves (Boston Women's Health Book Collective), 14
Ovarian cancer, 90-92
  risk of, 91-92
  survival rate, 92
  treatment of, 92-93
Ovariectomy, 21
Ovaries, 10, 11, 16, 18, 21, 51, 52
  removal of, 12
Ovulation, 18
Ovulatory cycles, 24

Palpitations, 13
Pancreas gland, 52
Papanicolaou, George, 82

Papanicolaou (Pap) smear, 26, 62, 64, 82, 85, 89
Parathyroid gland, 52
Partial hysterectomy, 94
Pelvic relaxation, 80-82
Penis, stimulation techniques, 123-124
Perimenopausal years, 18
Pessary, 29
Phenol, 165, 166
Physique, changes in, 31-32
Pins and needles (symptom), 13
Pituitary gland, 10, 23
Polyps, 78-80
  prognosis for, 79-80
Postmenopause, 11, 18
Pre-menopausal years, 18
Progesterone, 25, 53, 55, 57, 77, 79, 89
  production of, 10, 52, 54
Prostheses, 109
Psychosexual therapy, 128
Psychosomatic Medicine, 8
Psychotherapy, 45-46
Puberty, estrogen and, 53-54

Radiation therapy, 87
Radical hysterectomy, 72
"Rap groups," 44-45
Rectocele (rectal descent), 28
Refactory period, male, 122
Relaxation, 160-162
  exercises for, 161
Resource directory, 201-245
  employment, 229-235
  free breast examination, 220-221
  publications, 214-220, 222-229, 236-237
  beauty care, 217-218
  cancer and surgery, 218-220

Resource directory (cont.)
   educational directories, 227–229
   emotional well-being, 222–223
   exercise and diet, 216–217
   for lesbians, 225–227
   for living alone, 223–224
   on sexuality, 224–225
   reading list, 240–245
     fiction, 244–245
     general sourcebooks, 245
     journal, 244
     nonfiction, 240–244
   women's organizations, 238–240
Reuben, David, 16–17
Rhythm method, 25
Ricks, D. F., 133
Rockefeller, Happy, 82
Roosevelt, Franklin D., 4
Ruebsaat, Helmut J., 131, 138

Scarf, Maggie, 136
Secretions, cervical, 55
Self-esteem, 16
Self-image, 12
   sex at menopause and, 129
Self-indulgence, virtues of, 48–49
Senile vaginitis, 28
Sex:
   alternatives to marriage, 118–121
     finding new partner, 120–121
     homosexuality, 118
     involved but unmarried, 119–120
     living alone, 120
     older women, younger men, 118–119
   atrophy, preventing, 113
   attractiveness, 113–114
   basic physiology of, 121–122
   choices, 114–117
     celibacy, 115
     making, 114–115
     marriage, 116–117
   impotence in older men, 124
   making love to older man, 122–124
     stimulation techniques, 123–124
   self-image and, 129
   touching and kissing, 125–126
   transition period, 128–129
   use of fantasy, 125
Sex therapy, 127–128, 142–143
Shore, Miles, 139
Silicone implants, 168
Skin care, 170–171
   improving through surgery, 165–169
     altering facial features, 167
     for the body, 168–169
     for the breast, 168
     cryosurgery, 166–167
     dermabrasion, 167
     dermaplaning, 166
     face-lifts, 167–168
     face peels, 165–166
   nutrition and, 170
Sleeplessness, 13
Smoking, 145, 171
Spinnbarkeit phenomenon, 55
Sterilization, 25
Stillman, Irwin, 152
Stress, 5–6, 29
Stress amenorrhea, 23
Surgical menopause, 12, 21–22
Symptoms, menopausal, 12–13, 16
   changes and, 18–34
     abnormal bleeding, 25–26
     atrophic changes, 26–29
     body and physique, 31–32

constipation, 33
contraception, 24-25
depression, 31
headaches, 33
hot flushes, 33
insomnia, 33
osteoporosis, 30-31
physician's help, 19-20
regular checkups, 33-34
sex drive, 33
surgical menopause, 21-22
vasomotor instability, 22-24
endometriosis, 76-77
estrogen production and, 56-57
male menopause, 131

Tension and relaxation, 160-162
exercises, 161
Testosterone, 143
Testosterone replacement therapy, 124
Therapeutic ablation, 111
Therapists:
how to find, 46
judging effectiveness of, 47
Therapy, 45-47
"total push" approach, 46
Thermography, 103-104
Thighs, surgical correction of, 168
Thomas, Dylan, 135
Thompson, Clara, 7
Thrombophlebitis, 60
Through Navaho Eyes (Worth and Adair), 135-136
Thyroid gland, 52
Tiredness, 13, 20
Touching, sexual, 125-126

U.S. Department of Health, Education, and Welfare, 87

U.S. National Center for Health Statistics, 144
University of Chicago, 8
Urethra, the, 28
Urethral inflammations, 28
Urethrocele (descent of the urethra into the vagina), 28
Urinary pregnancy test, 26
Urinary tract infections, 28
Urination, frequent, 29
Uterine fibroids, 70
Uterus, 21, 28, 53, 72,
endometriosis, 75-78

Vaginal bleeding, 15, 18, 21, 62
Vaginal creams, 28
Vaginal discharge, 28
Vaginal infections, 25
Vaginitis, 26
Valium, 12
Vaseline, 113, 128
Vasomotor instability, 22-24
Veins, surgical correction of, 169
Vibrators, 124
Vitamin A, 170
Vitamin B-complex, 148, 170
Vitamin C, 170
Vitamin D, 148, 154

Waist, surgical correction of, 168
Weideger, Paula, 7
Weight, 145-146
changes in calorie needs, 146-147
desirable (for women of ages 25 and over), 146
See also Diet
West Germany, 9, 13
Worth, Sol, 135-136
Wright, Frank Lloyd, 135
Wrinkles, surgical correction of, 169

Wrinkling of the skin, 32

X chromosomes, 53
Xerography (or xeroradiography), 103
X-ray radiation, 104
X-rays, 30, 79, 80–81, 88, 93, 100, 105
 of the breasts, 102–103

Yoga, 156
Youth cult, 40–41
YWCAs, 45, 156

Zilbach, Joan, 141